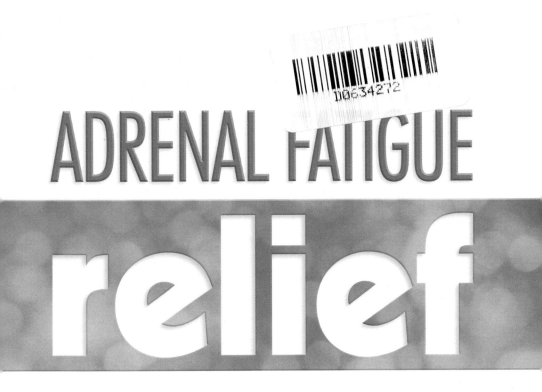

ADRENAL FATIGUE

relief

REGAIN ENERGY, REDUCE STRESS, RECLAIM YOUR LIFE

Sorrel Davis

Healthy Living Publications
Summertown, Tennessee

Library of Congress Cataloging-in-Publication Data

Names: Davis, Sorrel, author.
Title: Adrenal fatigue relief : regain energy, reduce stress, reclaim your life /
    Sorrel Davis.
Description: Summertown, Tennessee : Healthy Living Publications, [2018] |
    Includes bibliographical references and index.
Identifiers: LCCN 2017053545 (print) | LCCN 2017054645 (ebook) | ISBN
    9781570678462 (e-book) | ISBN 9781570673535 (paperback)
Subjects: LCSH: Adrenal glands—Diseases—Treatment—Popular works. |
    Self-care, Health.
Classification: LCC RC659 (ebook) | LCC RC659 .D38 2018 (print) | DDC
    616.4/5—dc23
LC record available at https://lccn.loc.gov/2017053545

Book Publishing CO.

We chose to print this title on responsibly harvested paper stock
certified by the Forest Stewardship Council,® an independent
auditor of responsible forestry practices. For more information,
visit us.fsc.org.

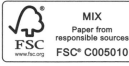

MIX
Paper from
responsible sources
FSC® C005010

Cover and interior design: John Wincek
Stock photography: 123 RF

Printed in the United States of America

Healthy Living Publications
a division of Book Publishing Company
PO Box 99
Summertown, TN 38483
888-260-8458
bookpubco.com

ISBN: 978-1-57067-353-5

Disclaimer: The information in this book
is presented for educational purposes only.
It isn't intended to be a substitute for the
medical advice of a physician, dietitian, or
other health-care professional.

23 22 21 20 19 18   1 2 3 4 5 6 7 8 9

CONTENTS

PREFACE

I n 1998 James L. Wilson coined the term "adrenal fatigue" to identify a condition that he believes is the consequence of ongoing stress: below-optimal adrenal function. He devised this term to put a name to the cluster of common symptoms that he asserts are caused by modern stress and to distinguish it from Addison's disease, a serious, long-term endocrine disorder. But many doctors say these symptoms can be due to other health problems or that the "symptoms" are merely very common complaints experienced by people in general. Who is right?

Wilson's credentials are impressive: He has three doctorates and two master's degrees in a variety of health-related disciplines, including nutrition, chiropractic medicine, and naturopathic medicine. He was also one of the founding members of the Canadian College of Naturopathic Medicine, the institution where he obtained his degree.

After conceiving the term, Wilson proceeded to create an empire of exclusive protocols to diagnose the condition, along with supplements specifically formulated to treat it. People who had long been suffering with the numerous symptoms that Wilson claims are indicators of "adrenal fatigue" latched onto this label and to his methods in a desperate attempt to find relief. Wilson claims to have successfully treated thousands of patients throughout North Amer-

War will never cease until babies begin to come into the world with larger cerebrums and smaller adrenal glands

H. L. MENCKEN (1880–1956)
American journalist, satirist, and cultural critic

iv

ica, and his proprietary supplements have been sold in numerous countries throughout the world.

Still, many questions remain. Is adrenal fatigue a true medical condition, or is it something simply construed by a well-meaning but misguided individual? Is it physiologically possible for the adrenal glands to malfunction or become depleted due to excessive stress? What tests are available to confirm a diagnosis of "adrenal fatigue"? And what treatment methods are medically endorsed and scientifically proven to alleviate the symptoms associated with it?

The answers to these questions and more are covered in the following pages. You'll take a tour of the adrenal glands, learn what makes the adrenals tick, and discover what can cause them to fail. You'll also read about disorders of the adrenal glands, explore the types of tests that are available to check for these disorders, and delve into the controversies surrounding "adrenal fatigue." In addition, you'll learn about the medically confirmed health consequences of prolonged stress and discover safe, inexpensive (or free!) time-tested strategies that will help you feel better, reduce your overall stress levels, and gain more energy. Equipped with this information, you will finally be able to take charge of your symptoms, reclaim your health, and take back your life. Your future is waiting . . . just turn the page!

Sorrel Davis

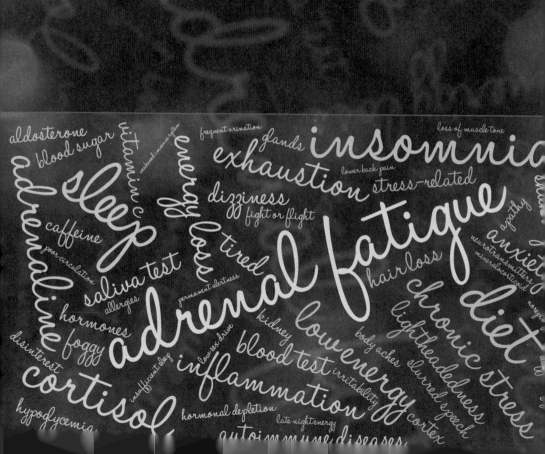

ADRENAL FATIGUE

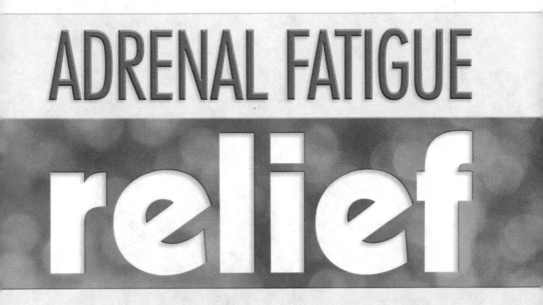

relief

REGAIN ENERGY, REDUCE STRESS, RECLAIM YOUR LIFE

1

Evolution has meant that
our prefrontal lobes are too small,
our adrenal glands are too big,
and our reproductive organs
apparently designed by committee;
a recipe which, alone or in combination,
is very certain to lead to
some unhappiness and disorder.

CHRISTOPHER HITCHENS (1949–2011)
American author, columnist,
and social critic

The Birth of "Adrenal Fatigue"

T he term "adrenal fatigue" was coined in 1998 by chiropractor and naturopath James Wilson. Since then it has been widely employed by alternative health-care providers, the media, and the general public to describe an alleged condition caused by chronic exposure to stressful situations. The body's reactions to stress are associated with an enhanced secretion of a number of hormones, such as adrenaline and cortisol, the effect of which is to increase mobilization of energy sources and adapt the individual to its new circumstance. The adrenal glands—small organs located above the kidneys—help the body cope with stress by producing these so-called stress hormones.

Supporters of adrenal fatigue believe the condition begins when the various stressors of life overwhelm the body and become too much for it to handle. According to the theory of adrenal fatigue, when people are confronted with ongoing stress for long periods of time, their adrenal glands are unable to keep up with the body's demand for these stress hormones. When that occurs, symptoms of "adrenal fatigue" begin to surface.

Wilson not only conceived the term for the disorder but he also invented exclusive diagnosis and treatment protocols, positioning himself as the premiere expert, diagnostician, and practitioner to both identify and cure the condition. In addition, Wilson developed specific tests and supplements as well as an education and training program for other practitioners of his protocols who are eligible

3

for wholesale supplement discounts, clinical support, and patient referrals. Despite the fact that Wilson's protocols have no medical endorsement or scientific proof, his theories and methods have proliferated worldwide.

Because stress is at the heart of supposed adrenal fatigue, any discussion pertaining to it must begin with a basic understanding of stress and the stress-coping mechanisms of the body. Everybody knows what stress is, or thinks they do, since we've all experienced it at one time or another. Stress is basically an unavoidable consequence of contemporary life, and it could justifiably be deemed the "disease" of the twenty-first century. Although we all have encountered stress, most people would be hard pressed to define exactly what it is.

At its core, stress is a physiological (condition of the body) state with psychological (mental/emotional) components that is produced by a change in the environment (i.e., a stressor) that disrupts the body's internal balance, known as physiological homeostasis. "Stress" could be described as any situation that tends to disturb the equilibrium between a living organism and its environment. In day-to-day life, we encounter a variety of stressful situations, such as job pressure, examinations, psychosocial stress, and physical stresses due to trauma, surgery, and various medical disorders. Regardless of the nature of the stressor, and regardless of whether it's real or simply perceived as real, the goal of the body's stress-management systems is always the same: to adapt to the change. How well the body adapts and equalizes depends on a variety of factors: a person's age, health, sex, nutritional status, and genetic makeup. Of course, many of these factors are difficult if not impossible to modify or control.

The term "stress" as we currently interpret it is credited to János Hugo Bruno "Hans" Selye (1907–1982), who is considered the father of modern stress research. Selye, an Austrian-Canadian endocrinologist of Hungarian descent, gained international recognition for introducing the concept of stress in a medical context. He was the first physician to connect perceived stressful events in the environment to human biological responses. Selye showed that persistent stress caused various diseases in laboratory animals, including heart attack, kidney disease, rheumatoid arthritis, and stroke. This was groundbreaking, because it demonstrated for the first time that stress might be responsible for a broad range of unrelated human diseases.

Most people associate stress with distress, and any favorable connotations of stress are generally disregarded. But a full definition of stress must also include "good" stress, or what Selye termed "eustress." This positive type of stress results in the release of feel-good chemicals called endorphins that can actually have a beneficial influence on emotional as well as physical well-being.

General Adaptation Syndrome

In 1936 Selye created the stress model known as general adaptation syndrome (GAS), which explains how the body adapts to external stressors in a predictable pattern so homeostasis can be reestablished and maintained. To do this, the body relies in large part on its hormonal "stress response" system. But Selye discovered that the body has a finite supply of energy to adapt to stressors, and that its systems can become overburdened and compromised when exposure to a stressor is continuous. Selye's GAS model is made up of three stages that reflect what the body goes through in response to stress: (1) alarm, (2) resistance, and (3) exhaustion.

1. **Alarm.** The sympathetic ("fight or flight") nervous system is activated at this stage, which initiates the release of "stress hormones," such as adrenaline and cortisol. People in the throes of the alarm stage will have muscle tension, a faster pulse and respiration rate, and increased perspiration. They may seem anxious or agitated and may have gastrointestinal disturbances and trouble sleeping.

2. **Resistance.** After the stressful event concludes, the parasympathetic ("rest and digest") nervous system returns many of the body's functions back to normal. Although the affected person may outwardly appear "normal," adrenaline and cortisol are still circulating at higher-than-normal levels, and the body is still on red alert. This stage can cause someone to feel anxious, depressed, or fatigued.

3. **Exhaustion.** If the stress has persisted for a long period, a person will reach the exhaustion stage. At this point the individual will suffer enormous mental, physical, and emotional repercussions with potentially serious psychological and physiological consequences that could result in illness or even death. Although this stage is the most critical, it's also the most rare.

Attempting to Define the Elusive

Selye's efforts were considered radical at the time and were initially met with professional skepticism. But his unprecedented ideas about stress, along with his scientific diligence and persistence, eventually garnered the respect of his peers and birthed an entirely new field of medicine—the study of biological stress and its effects. Today the field has mushroomed and now includes the work of thousands of researchers who continue to make advances in the field of stress research by studying the connections between stress and illness.

Nevertheless, because the experience of stress is highly subjective, it's almost impossible to define it within a medical framework. If a medical phenomenon can't be accurately defined, it also can't be accurately measured. And if it can't be accurately measured, it can't be quantified, which makes it a challenge to observe and research it scientifically.

Complicating matters further is the fact that stress can be both positive and healthy (eustress)—as occurs with favorable situations, such as getting married, starting a new job, or buying a house—or negative and harmful (distress), which is how we most commonly define it. In addition, what one person perceives as a stressful event may be exciting or even dull to another person depending on a variety of uniquely individual factors, such as personality, physical strength, age, gender, life experiences, genetic makeup, or general health.

Although scientists agree that a degree of stress is a normal part of responding to changes in our physical and social environments, most people focus on the negative feelings stress produces, even though positive events can generate stress as well. In a medical or biological context, stress can be defined as any physical, mental, or emotional factor that causes tension in the body or mind. It can be triggered by any incident that an individual believes threatens his or her mental, physical, or financial resources, whether the stressor is external (coming from outside the body) or internal (psychological or disease states), or whether that stress arises from positive or negative circumstances.

Stress-related health conditions are a common consequence of excessive and prolonged demands on a person's coping reserves. In general, there are three different types of stress: (1) acute stress, which is associated with the fight-or-flight response; (2) chronic stress, which is typically associated with the challenges of daily life; and (3) eustress, which is the result of positive experiences.

The Physiological Effects of Stress

While it's fairly obvious that excessive stress can negatively affect coping skills and impair a person's ability to manage the activities of daily living, the effect stress has on the various systems, organs, and tissues of the body are less apparent but equally significant. The following list shows how some of the key body systems respond to stress:

Nervous system. When the body is under stress, the sympathetic nervous system activates the fight-or-flight response. This triggers the release of "stress hormones," such as adrenaline and cortisol, from the adrenal glands. These hormones elevate heart rate, raise blood pressure, increase blood glucose levels, and interfere with digestive processes.

Musculoskeletal system. When the body is under stress, muscles tense and become more rigid, potentially triggering headaches, neck and back pain, and a variety of musculoskeletal problems.

Respiratory system. Stress can cause hyperventilation, which may lead to abnormal loss of carbon dioxide from the blood and which in turn can trigger panic attacks.

Cardiovascular system. Stress that's extreme but temporary causes an increase in heart rate, stronger contractions of the heart muscle, and dilation of blood vessels that direct blood to the heart. Repeated episodes can inflame the coronary arteries and may contribute to heart attack.

Endocrine system. When the body is under stress, the brain sends signals from the hypothalamus to the adrenal glands to produce epinephrine, which triggers the liver to produce more glucose.

Gastrointestinal system. Stress can cause heartburn or acid reflux and, in extreme cases, nausea and vomiting. It can impair nutrient absorption and digestion and may trigger either constipation or diarrhea. It can also cause loss of appetite or provoke overeating.

Reproductive system. Stress can induce irregular menstrual cycles and more painful periods in women. It can also decrease libido (sexual desire) in both men and women.

Common Signs and Symptoms of Stress

Our bodies are designed to handle small doses of stress, but we aren't equipped to handle long-term, chronic stress without harmful consequences. In addition to the physiological repercussions outlined above, stress can affect general physical health and all areas of life, including behavior, emotions, mood, and the ability to think clearly. Symptoms of many preexisting medical conditions may also worsen during times of stress. There is virtually no part of the body that's immune to it.

Sometimes people become so accustomed to living with stress that they don't know how to identify it and aren't fully aware of its specific effects on them. Here are just a few of the countless warning signs that stress is wreaking havoc on a person's body and mind:

- acid reflux
- chest pain
- confusion
- constipation
- depression
- diarrhea
- difficulty breathing
- excessive sweating
- fatigue
- frequent headaches
- frequent urination
- heartburn

- increased anger and hostility
- jaw clenching
- loss of appetite
- low energy
- muscle spasms
- nausea
- overeating
- poor judgment
- racing thoughts
- sleep changes (too much or not enough)
- stomach pain
- suicidal thoughts
- tremors
- wild mood swings

The Evolution of Stress and Health

Today's stress differs greatly not only from what our evolutionary ancestors faced but also from what our ancestors of just the past century or two experienced. Over the course of human evolution, the stress response has helped the human species survive and deal with environmental challenges by supplying physiological coping mechanisms that imparted the energy and quick-thinking skills needed to fight off attackers or escape deadly situations.

Contrarily, contemporary stress mostly originates from the ongoing pressures of daily living as well as fear and worry about what *might* happen in the future, and yet our bodies respond in the same ways as those of our prehistoric predecessors. When the stress response is constantly being engaged, it regularly floods the body with stress hormones and taxes the normal functioning of the body's systems. Modern stress is often chronic and typically arises from circumstances over which we have little control. Our response to it has become ingrained and habituated, but in most instances it provides no benefit to us. Instead, this ceaseless, acculturated stress has been implicated as a primary contributor to an impressive array of "twenty-first-century diseases," including anxiety, cancer, depression, high blood pressure, gastrointestinal dysfunction, neurological disorders (such as Parkinson's disease), immune system disorders (including multiple sclerosis and rheumatoid arthritis), stroke, and many others. In fact, it's difficult to think of a condition that stress doesn't instigate or aggravate to one degree or another, and a growing number of researchers have come to believe that stress could actually be the genesis of all modern disease.

Could It Be the Vagus Nerve?

The vagus nerve is the longest cranial nerve in the body. The word "vagus" is Latin for "wandering," and the nerve was so named because its path in the body is long and circuitous. The tone (health and vibrancy) of the vagus nerve is key to activating the parasympathetic ("rest and digest") nervous system. Vagal tone is measured by tracking heart rate alongside breathing rate, which is known as heart rate variability (HRV). Heart rate increases slightly when we inhale, and it slows down slightly when we exhale. The greater the difference between the inhalation heart rate and the exhalation heart rate, the higher (healthier) the vagal tone. A higher vagal-tone frequency means the body can relax more quickly after a stressful event.

The vagus nerve regulates the digestive system and also affects the cardiovascular, endocrine, immune, and respiratory systems. In addition, the vagus nerve innervates the gut, kidneys, liver, lungs, and spleen. The vagus nerve provides a bidirectional link between the gut and the brain and connects all the major organs (excluding the adrenal glands and thyroid). Not surprisingly, the proper functioning of the vagus nerve is crucial for both physical and mental well-being. Although the vagus nerve isn't the only nerve in the parasympathetic nervous system, it's by far the most important because it has the most far-reaching effects.

Vagus nerve dysfunction (when the vagus nerve is either overactive or underactive) can result in the manifestation of a wide range of symptoms. For example, an underactive vagus nerve can lead to delayed gastric emptying (gastroparesis). That's because peristalsis (the involuntary constriction and relaxation of the muscles of the intestine) is under the control of the vagus nerve, and any damage to the vagus nerve will impede gut motility. When the vagus nerve is hyperactive, it can result in an abnormally low heart rate (bradycardia), temporary loss of consciousness (syncope), and a variety of other symptoms.

Healthy vagus nerve activity promotes relaxation, lowers heart rate, decreases anxiety, and reduces depression. Higher vagal tone is associated with better mood and greater resilience to stress. Conversely, vagus nerve dysfunction or a low vagal tone is associated with increased heart rate, elevated blood pressure, heightened stress response, cognitive impairment, and poor digestion. The vagus nerve plays a role in almost every disease that involves hyperarousal, such as anxiety, epilepsy, heart attack, high blood pressure, inflammation, insomnia, panic disorder, and post-traumatic stress disorder (PTSD). The vagus nerve has also been implicated in tinnitus (ringing in the ears) and, not surprisingly, irritable bowel syndrome (IBS).

Because the vagus nerve interfaces with the parasympathetic nervous system, its health and activity influence the following body functions:

DECREASES	INCREASES	REGULATES
heart rate	gastrointestinal peristalsis	glucose homeostasis
inflammation	satiety from food	insulin secretion
neural (relating to the nerves or nervous system) processes	neurogenesis (the growth and development of nerves and nervous tissue)	
sweating		

Vagus nerve stimulation counterbalances the stress response of the sympathetic nervous system and normalizes HPA axis dysregulation, decreasing heart rate and promoting healthy digestion and relaxation. It also has an antidepressant effect and helps keep inflammation in check. Increased vagal tone is linked with greater intimacy and social bonding, whereas diminished vagal tone is associated with negative moods, loneliness, and social isolation.

Pain is one of the most common symptoms of vagus nerve dysfunction. Often the pain is accompanied by muscle cramps on moving. The pain can be so severe that it may interfere with the ability to walk. Vagus nerve damage or dysfunction can inhibit swallowing and impair the normal gag reflex. Because the vagus nerve controls some of the muscles in the throat, damage to the vagus nerve can also alter a person's voice.

The connection between anxiety and the vagus nerve is well established. When functioning properly, the vagus nerve opposes the sympathetic fight-or-flight response. Dysfunction of the vagus nerve, however, leaves the sympathetic response unopposed, leading to anxiety, depression, hyperarousal, increased heart rate, and insomnia.

Vagus nerve stimulation (VNS) refers to any technique that stimulates the vagus nerve, including manual or electrical stimulation. It was first observed in the 1880s that manual massage and compression of the carotid artery in the cervical region of the neck could suppress seizures, an effect attributable to rudimentary stimulation of the vagus nerve. Electrical VNS studies were conducted during the 1930s and 1940s to understand the influence of the autonomic nervous system on modulating brain activity, and subsequent studies confirmed the anticonvulsant effects of VNS on seizures. Various forms of paced breathing can also influence the brain's electrical activity, which might be mediated by vagus nerve stimulation arising from the diaphragm. This type of cardio-respiratory stimulation of the vagus nerve helps explain some of the positive emotional and cognitive benefits of aerobic exercise, deep breathing, and yoga.

Dedicated clinical trials eventually led to approval in 1997 by the United States Food and Drug Administration (FDA) of an implanted VNS device for the treatment of refractory epilepsy. Vagus nerve stimulation is also an FDA-approved therapy for treatment-resistant depression. Researchers are currently studying VNS as a potential treatment for a variety of other conditions, including Alzheimer's disease, migraine headache, and multiple sclerosis.

In conventional vagus nerve stimulation, a device is surgically implanted under the skin on the chest, and a wire is threaded under the skin to connect the device to the left vagus nerve. (The right vagus nerve isn't used because it carries fibers that supply nerves to the heart.) When the device is activated, it sends electrical signals along the vagus nerve to the brain stem, which then sends signals to certain areas of the brain.

Although vagus nerve stimulation can be invasive, new noninvasive methods, which don't require surgical implantation, are now available in the United States for episodic cluster headaches (a rare but extremely painful primary headache disorder characterized by recurrent unilateral attacks). Noninvasive VNS devices have also been approved for use in Europe to treat depression, epilepsy, and pain. Although these have not yet been approved for use in the United States, they are currently being studied.

Unless you have a surgically implanted VNS device, you can't actually stimulate the vagus nerve directly. However, because the vagus nerve passes through the facial muscles, inner ear, throat, lungs, diaphragm, and gut, you can indirectly stimulate it through certain practices that influence it via the mind-body feedback loop. The following are a few of these techniques that you can practice in the privacy of your own home. If you have asthma, heart disease, hearing problems, high or low blood pressure, or any other health conditions that might be exacerbated by these exercises, get clearance from your doctor or health-care provider before trying them.

CONSCIOUS BREATHING

Conscious breathing is the practice of breathing with awareness and intention. It's also one of the fastest and easiest ways to positively influence the state of the nervous system. The objective is to move the belly and diaphragm in conjunction with the breath and to slow down your breathing. Vagus nerve stimulation occurs when the breath is decreased to five to seven breaths per minute from the typical ten to fourteen breaths per minute. This can be achieved by inhaling to a count of 4, holding the breath for a count of 7, and exhaling to a count of 8. Breathe in slowly through your nose to a count of 4, allowing your lower belly to rise as you fill your lungs. Let your inhalation completely fill your lungs, gently and naturally expanding your lower abdomen, not your chest. Hold the breath for a count of 7. Then slowly exhale through your nose to a count of 8. Completely release the air during your exhalations, letting the abdomen naturally relax and deflate. To increase the benefits even more with your exhalation, put your tongue on the roof of your mouth (just behind your upper teeth), purse your lips slightly, and gently exhale through your mouth to a count of 8.

Start by practicing conscious breathing for six cycles per session. If you like, you can gradually work your way up to twelve cycles or more per session. Conscious breathing will be most effective if it is practiced daily, with at least one or two sessions per day.

Although ideally you should be seated with your back straight, your feet flat on the floor, and your hands resting comfortably in your lap, you can practice conscious breathing in any place or circumstance, including lying down (try it just before you go to sleep) and during times of stress. When used regularly, it will help you develop the skill of relaxation, even in challenging situations.

OCEAN BREATH

You can further stimulate the vagus nerve when you practice conscious breathing (see above) by creating a slight constriction at the back of your throat and creating an "ahhh" sound with your mouth closed. Then breathe out as though you are fogging up a mirror, again keeping your mouth closed and silently saying "ahhh" as you exhale. You will notice your breath making an "ocean" sound, softly moving in and out, like ocean waves. The breath should be steady, rhythmic, smooth, and full. Let your inhalations expand your lungs fully, then completely release the air during your exhalations. Direct the breath to travel over your vocal cords and across the back of your throat. Keep your mouth closed but your lips soft and relaxed. Concentrate on the sound of your breath and let the "ocean" sound soothe your mind. It should be audible to you, but not so loud that someone standing several feet away can hear it.

Start by practicing ocean breath for six cycles per session. If you like, you can gradually work your way up to twelve cycles or more per session. Ocean breath will be most effective if it is practiced daily, with at least one or two sessions per day.

HUMMING OR CHANTING

The vagus nerve has branches that run from the brain stem to the larynx (voice box), and it's responsible for controlling the movement of the vocal cords. In fact, damage to the vagus nerve is the specific cause of vocal cord paralysis. Stimulating the vagus nerve through the vibrations of humming is an easy and enjoyable way to influence the health of the nervous system. All you have to do is choose a favorite melody! If you prefer, you can chant the word "OM," "home," "hum," or just "hmmm," stretching out the "mmm" sound as long as you can. Observe and enjoy the sensations in your chest, throat, lips, and head. This is an excellent exercise to do when you're alone in the car and are stuck in traffic or are at a stoplight. You can practice humming or chanting for a few minutes at a time or for 15 to 20 minutes per session, with up to two sessions per day. The exercise will be most effective if it's done on a daily basis.

SINGING

Singing loudly increases oxytocin (see page 44), as well as works the muscles in the back of the throat to activate the vagus nerve. Singing, whether it's in unison (as with a choir or group of friends) or alone, will stimulate vagus nerve function, increase relaxation, and elevate mood.

VALSALVA MANEUVER

This is a rather simple exercise with a complicated-sounding name. It involves gently attempting to exhale against a closed airway, which increases the pressure inside the chest cavity and improves vagal tone. Sit comfortably with your feet flat on the floor and your back straight. Take a deep breath through your nose, keep your mouth closed, pinch your nose with your thumb and index finger, and very gently attempt to breathe out. Do not use any force whatsoever. Keep your cheek muscles tight; don't allow them to bulge out. Do this for about five seconds, then exhale completely through your nose. Do the exercise three times per session, two or three times per day.

DIVING REFLEX

The diving reflex is a complex cardiovascular-respiratory response to immersion. It slows the heart rate, increases blood flow to the brain, relaxes the body, and reduces anger. Splashing very cold water on your face from your chin to your scalp and covering both cheeks is all that's needed to induce the diving reflex. Alternatively, you can cool down the nervous system by putting ice cubes in a zip-lock bag, sealing the bag, and holding the ice against your face while briefly holding your breath.

EXPOSURE TO COLD

Studies show that when the body adjusts to cold, the fight-or-flight response (sympathetic nervous system) decreases, and the "rest and digest" response (parasympathetic nervous system) increases. All of this is mediated by the vagus nerve. Just drinking cold water or splashing cold water on your face (see "Diving Reflex" above) may be enough to stimulate your vagus nerve. You can also take cold showers, finish a warm shower with thirty seconds of ice-cold water, or take a swim in an unheated pool.

MASSAGE

Research shows that massage can stimulate the vagus nerve, increasing vagal activity and vagal tone. The vagus nerve can also be stimulated by massaging specific areas of the body, such as the feet (reflexology) or neck. A neck massage along the carotid sinus (the right side of the throat near where you check your pulse) can also stimulate the vagus nerve.

PROBIOTICS

The presence of healthy bacteria in the gut creates a positive feedback loop through the vagus nerve, increasing its tone. Studies have shown that supplementing with *Lactobacillus rhamnosus* (*L. rhamnosus*), a particular probiotic strain, promotes various positive changes in gamma-aminobutyric acid (GABA), one of the body's primary neurotransmitters that's mediated by the vagus nerve and acts to calm the central nervous system.

THERAPEUTIC FASTING OR CALORIE REDUCTION

The vagus nerve is responsible for regulating digestion. When the body is under duress, the digestive system shuts down. During a fast, an empty stomach sends signals to the brain that digestion is unnecessary, so energy resources can be used for relaxation instead. Intermittent fasting or reducing caloric intake within a limited time frame will increase high-frequency heart rate variability, the measurement of vagal tone (see page 10).

HUMOR THERAPY

Laughter relaxes the entire body and has positive effects on the "rest and digest" (parasympathetic) nervous system. The process of laughing increases abdominal pressure and diaphragmatic movement. Because the vagus nerve passes through the diaphragm, these movements provide vagal stimulation and send a signal through the nerve telling the body to relax. In addition, laughter reduces the level of stress hormones and triggers the release of mood-enhancing hormones, such as endorphins, which are the body's natural painkillers. Find something in your workplace or daily activities that makes you smile, and actively seek out stimuli that make you laugh and that you can access anytime throughout the day. You can also watch humorous movies or television shows, read humorous books, go to a comedy club, or simply joke around with friends. Some health providers incorporate humor therapy as part of their treatment protocols. You don't even have to laugh out loud to experience the soothing benefits of laughter. Finding something funny that makes you chuckle on the inside tends to be just as therapeutic.

2

Trying to describe a good marriage
is like trying to describe
your adrenal glands.
You know they're in there functioning,
but you don't really understand
how they work.

HELEN GURLEY BROWN (1922–2012)
American author and publisher

The Essential Adrenals

he adrenal glands, also known as suprarenal glands, are small, walnut-sized, triangular-shaped glands located on the top of both kidneys. Their name correlates to their location in the body: *ad*, meaning "near" or "at," and *renes*, meaning "kidneys." Surprisingly, the glands aren't symmetrical. The right adrenal gland is triangular, and the left adrenal gland is shaped more like a half-moon. They each have a yellowish hue and are about two and a half inches in length and one inch wide.

The adrenals have three distinct components: the adipose capsule, the cortex, and the medulla. The capsule is a protective layer of fat that surrounds each gland. Although this layer isn't technically part of the glands themselves, its purpose is to enclose and protect each of the adrenals. The adrenal cortex is the outer region and comprises about 80 percent of the volume of the gland. It fully surrounds the adrenal medulla, which sits in the center. The adrenal cortex is composed of three individual zones that perform slightly different functions. Starting from the outside, they are the zona glomerulosa, the zona fasciculata, and the zona reticularis. The innermost region of the adrenal gland is the medulla. It's surrounded by the adrenal cortex and comprises only 20 percent of the gland's volume. Unlike the cortex, the medulla does not have separate zones.

The role of the adrenal glands is to release certain hormones, many of which have to do with how the body responds to stress, directly into the bloodstream. As discussed in chapter one, stress can be broadly defined as any stimulus (stressor) that disrupts the body's internal balance (physiological homeostasis). Although there is some interaction between the adrenal cortex and the adrenal medulla, each performs distinct and separate functions and secretes specific hormones. One of the primary differences between them is that the hormones released by the adrenal cortex are essential to life and those secreted by the adrenal medulla are not.

Adrenal Cortex

The adrenal cortex produces two main groups of corticosteroid hormones: glucocorticoids and mineralocorticoids. The release of glucocorticoids is triggered by the hypothalamus (see page 42) and pituitary gland (see page 45), and mineralocorticoids are mediated by signals triggered by the kidneys. The glucocorticoids have anti-inflammatory activity and are involved in the metabolism of carbohydrates, proteins, and fats, whereas the mineralocorticoids regulate the balance of salt and water in the body.

Hydrocortisone. Frequently referred to as cortisol, this glucocorticoid is believed to have hundreds of effects in the body. Cortisol's most important job is to help the body respond to stress, giving it a boost of energy so it can better handle a crisis. In addition, it helps maintain blood pressure and cardiovascular function, slows the immune system's inflammatory response, balances the effects of insulin in breaking down sugar for energy, and regulates the metabolism of proteins, carbohydrates, and fats. Cortisol also controls the body's circadian rhythm, commonly known as the sleep-wake cycle.

Because cortisol is so critical to health, the amount of it that's produced by the adrenal glands is carefully balanced. As with many other hormones, cortisol is regulated by the brain's hypothalamus and the pituitary gland, a pea-sized organ at the base of the brain.

For the adrenal cortex to produce cortisol, the hypothalamus must produce corticotropin-releasing hormone (CRH), which stimulates the pituitary gland to secrete adrenocorticotropic hormone (ACTH). In response, ACTH stimulates the adrenal glands to make and release cortisol hormones into the blood. In a healthy individual, both the hypothalamus and the pituitary gland will sense whether the blood has the right amount of cortisol in it. If there is too much or too little cortisol, these glands respectively change the amount of CRH and ACTH that gets released.

It's important to know that infection, trauma, excessive exercise, obesity, and debilitating disease can influence cortisol concentrations. Pregnancy, physical and emotional stress, and illness can increase cortisol levels. Cortisol levels may also increase as a result of hyperthyroidism (overactivity of the thyroid gland) or decrease due to hypothyroidism (underactivity of the thyroid gland). A number of drugs can influence cortisol levels, particularly oral contraceptives (birth control pills), hydrocortisone (the synthetic form of cortisol), and spironolactone, a steroid derivative that promotes sodium excretion and is used in the treatment of certain types of edema (swelling caused by excess fluid trapped in the body's tissues) and hypertension (high blood pressure). Note that adults have slightly higher cortisol levels than do children.

Aldosterone. The principal mineralocorticoid, aldosterone plays a central role in regulating blood pressure and certain electrolytes (sodium and potassium). It signals the kidneys to increase the amount of sodium the body sends into the bloodstream and to release more potassium into the urine, thereby helping to regulate the blood's pH level by controlling the amount of electrolytes in the blood. When aldosterone production falls too low, the kidneys aren't able to regulate salt and water balance, causing hypovolemia (a decrease in blood volume) and hypotension (a drop in blood pressure).

Corticosterone. This glucocorticoid works with hydrocortisone to regulate the immune response and suppress inflammatory reactions.

DHEA and androgenic steroids. This group of substances, called adrenal androgens, is released by the adrenal cortex and includes weak male sex hormones, notably dehydroepiandrosterone (DHEA) and testosterone. These are precursor hormones that are converted in the ovaries into female hormones (estrogens) and in the testes into male hormones (androgens). However, estrogens and androgens are produced in much larger amounts directly by the ovaries and testes.

In addition, adrenocorticotropic hormone (ACTH), secreted by the pituitary gland, stimulates the adrenal cortex, affecting the release of glucocorticoids, adrenal androgens, and, to a lesser extent, aldosterone.

Adrenal Medulla

Although the adrenal medulla doesn't affect any vital life functions, it's nonetheless important. The hormones epinephrine and norepinephrine (known as catecholamines) are produced by the adrenal medulla and are released after the sympathetic nervous system (see page 128) is stimulated, which occurs during periods of acute or chronic stress. This can result in the well-known fight-or-flight response—a process initiated when a person encounters a threatening or highly stressful situation.

Epinephrine. Commonly known as adrenaline, this hormone is secreted by the adrenal medulla in response to low blood levels of glucose or to physical or emotional stress. It increases heart rate, rushes blood to the muscles and brain, and spikes blood sugar levels by helping to convert glycogen to glucose in the liver. In addition, epinephrine facilitates the release of fatty acids from adipose (fat) tissue and causes dilation (widening) of the small arteries within muscle.

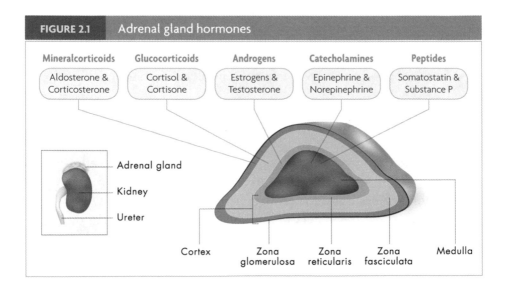

FIGURE 2.1   Adrenal gland hormones

Mineralcorticoids	Glucocorticoids	Androgens	Catecholamines	Peptides
Aldosterone & Corticosterone	Cortisol & Cortisone	Estrogens & Testosterone	Epinephrine & Norepinephrine	Somatostatin & Substance P

Adrenal gland
Kidney
Ureter

Cortex   Zona glomerulosa   Zona reticularis   Zona fasciculata   Medulla

Norepinephrine. Also called noradrenaline, this hormone works in conjunction with epinephrine in response to stress. However, it can cause blood vessels to narrow (known as vasoconstriction), resulting in high blood pressure.

Hypofunction (decreased or insufficient functioning) of the adrenal medulla is virtually unheard of. However, small vascular tumors, known as pheochromocytomas (see page 28), can arise within the adrenal medulla or elsewhere in the sympathetic nervous system. These tumors cause the irregular secretion of epinephrine and norepinephrine, which may lead to attacks of hypertension (elevated blood pressure), headache, heart palpitations, feelings of apprehension, sweating, flushing of the face, nausea, vomiting, and tingling of the extremities (arms and legs). Pheochromocytoma is equivalent to hyperfunction (excessive activity) of the adrenal medulla.

Disorders of the Adrenal Glands

ADRENAL INSUFFICIENCY

When the adrenal glands produce too little or too much of certain hormones, it can lead to hormonal imbalances and potentially serious or life-threatening health problems. Abnormalities in adrenal function may be caused by various diseases or disorders of the adrenal glands (primary adrenal insufficiency) or to inadequate secretion of ACTH by the pituitary gland (secondary adrenal insufficiency). Adrenal insufficiency usually develops gradually, but it can also appear suddenly, which is known as acute adrenal failure or adrenal crisis. If acute adrenal failure is left untreated, the consequences can be quite serious and may include coma, shock, seizures, and even death.

Primary Adrenal Insufficiency (Addison's Disease)

Addison's disease is a rare, life-threatening hormonal disorder that afflicts approximately one in ten thousand people annually. It occurs across all age groups and affects men and women equally. The condition is characterized by abdominal pain, depression, fatigue, low blood pressure, muscle weakness, nausea and vomiting, salt cravings, weight loss, and sometimes darkening of the skin. Addison's disease occurs when the adrenal glands don't produce enough of the hormone cortisol and, in some cases, the hormone aldosterone. For this reason the disease is sometimes referred to as chronic adrenal insufficiency or hypocortisolism.

Adrenal insufficiency was initially identified by English physician, researcher, and diagnostician Thomas Addison, who was the first to correlate a set of disease symptoms with pathological changes in one of the endocrine glands. During autopsies, Addison found that 70–90 percent of the cases had tuberculosis (TB). As the treatment for TB improved, the incidence of adrenal insufficiency due to TB greatly decreased. In developed countries today, TB is responsible for about 20 percent of the cases of primary adrenal insufficiency.

In about 70 percent of patients, Addison's disease is caused by the progressive destruction of the adrenal cortex (see page 20) by the body's own immune system. With autoimmune disorders, the immune system produces antibodies that attack the body's tissues or organs and gradually destroy them. Adrenal insufficiency occurs when at least 90 percent of the adrenal cortex has been destroyed, resulting in a deficiency of glucocorticoid and/or mineralocorticoid hormones. Occasionally only the adrenal glands are damaged, as with idiopathic adrenal insufficiency, but sometimes other glands are also affected, as with polyendocrine deficiency syndrome.

There are two separate forms of polyendocrine deficiency syndrome: type 1 and type 2. Type 1 occurs in children, and adrenal insufficiency may be accompanied by underactive parathyroid glands, depressed sexual development, pernicious anemia (a deficiency in the production of red blood cells through a lack of vitamin B_{12}), chronic candida infections, chronic active hepatitis, and in rare cases, alopecia (hair loss). Type 2, also known as Schmidt's syndrome, typically affects young adults. Symptoms of type 2 include an underactive thyroid gland, depressed sexual development, and diabetes mellitus. About 10 percent of people with type 2 polyendocrine deficiency syndrome have vitiligo, a condition in which pigment is lost from areas of the skin. Scientists believe that polyendocrine deficiency syndrome is inherited, because often other family members have one or more endocrine deficiencies.

Additional but less common causes of primary adrenal insufficiency include chronic infections (mainly fungal infections), cancer cells that

CAUSES OF ADRENAL INSUFFICIENCY

PRIMARY ADRENAL INSUFFICIENCY	SECONDARY ADRENAL INSUFFICIENCY
Anatomic destruction of the gland (acute or chronic):	**Hypothalamic-related insufficiency:**
Addison's disease (autoimmune adrenalitis; 85% of cases)	congenital
	corticotropin-releasing hormone (CRH) deficiency
hemorrhage	infiltration (the pathological accumulation in tissue or cells of substances not normal to them or in amounts in excess of the normal) or infection (hemochromatosis, lymphocytic hypophysitis, meningitis, sarcoidosis, TB)
infarction (obstruction of the blood supply to an organ or region of tissue)	
infections (TB, histoplasmosis, cryptococcosis, HIV, syphilis)	
invasion (the penetration of the body by a pathogenic microorganism or malignant cells in the body)	neoplasia (new and abnormal growth of tissue), primary or metastatic
	radiation therapy
surgical removal	surgery
trauma	trauma (fracture of the skull base)
Metabolic failure in hormone production:	**Suppression of the HPA axis:**
accelerated hepatic metabolism of cortisol	antipsychotic medication
adrenocorticotropic hormone (ACTH) or gluco-corticoid resistance	exogenous steroid administration
	steroid production from tumors
congenital adrenal hyperplasia	
cytotoxic agents	
enzyme inhibition	
Other causes:	**Pituitary:**
ACTH-blocking antibodies	congenital aplasia (the failure of an organ or tissue to develop or to function normally)
adrenal hypoplasia congenita	
familial adrenal insufficiency	infiltration (the pathological accumulation in tissue or cells of substances not normal to them or in amounts in excess of the normal) or infection (hemochromatosis, lymphocytic hypophysitis, meningitis, sarcoidosis, TB)
metabolic disorders	
mitochondrial disorders	
mutation in ACTH receptor gene	
	isolated ACTH deficiency
	radiation therapy
	surgery
	trauma
	tumors

spread to the adrenal glands from other parts of the body, amyloidosis (a rare disease that occurs when an abnormal protein called amyloid builds up in the body's organs), and surgical removal of the adrenal glands.

Secondary Adrenal Insufficiency

Secondary adrenal insufficiency occurs when there's a shortage of adrenocorticotropic hormone (ACTH), which causes a decrease in the production of cortisol but not aldosterone. The estimated prevalence is 150–280 people per million, with more women affected than men and a peak age of onset between fifty and sixty.

A temporary form of secondary adrenal insufficiency can occur when people who have been taking a glucocorticoid hormone, such as prednisone, for a long time suddenly stop or interrupt their regimen. Glucocorticoid hormones are commonly used to treat inflammatory illnesses, such as asthma, rheumatoid arthritis, and ulcerative colitis. They block the release of both corticotropin-releasing hormone (CRH) and ACTH. CRH signals the pituitary gland to release ACTH. If CRH levels drop, the pituitary gland doesn't receive any prompts to release ACTH, and as a result, the adrenals fail to secrete sufficient levels of cortisol.

Secondary adrenal insufficiency can also occur with the surgical removal of benign (noncancerous) ACTH-producing tumors of the pituitary gland (Cushing's disease). When the source of the ACTH (the tumor) is abruptly excised, replacement hormones must be administered until the normal production of ACTH and cortisol resumes. Cushing's disease is relatively rare, affecting ten to fifteen people out of every million each year. It most commonly affects adults between the ages of twenty and fifty, with women accounting for over 70 percent of the cases. Cushing's syndrome (as opposed to Cushing's disease) is a rare disorder resulting from prolonged exposure to excess glucocorticoids, regardless of the cause.

Although much less common, secondary adrenal insufficiency can ensue when the pituitary gland decreases in size or stops producing ACTH. This can be caused by tumors or infections in that area, radiation for the treatment of pituitary tumors, loss of blood flow to the pituitary gland, or surgical removal of parts of the hypothalamus or the pituitary gland.

OTHER DISEASES AND DISORDERS OF THE ADRENAL GLANDS

Congenital Adrenal Hyperplasia

Congenital adrenal hyperplasia (CAH) is an inherited form of adrenal insufficiency that is caused by mutations in the genetic coding for the essential enzymes needed to produce cortisol, aldosterone, or both. In its classical form, this disease appears in approximately 1 in 15,000 births. CAH is caused by a deficiency of an enzyme (adrenal steroid 21-hydroxylase) that's necessary for the synthesis of cortisol and aldosterone by the human body. In its severest form, classical CAH results in the uncontrolled loss of salt and fluids from the body, and if this condition goes undetected, it can lead to adrenal crisis and death.

A person must inherit a defective enzyme trait from each parent to become afflicted with CAH. (This is referred to as an autosomal recessive disease.) CAH affects males and females in equal numbers. For parents who have had a child affected with CAH, there is a 25 percent (one in four) chance of producing a second affected child. Prenatal diagnosis and prenatal treatment of a potentially affected fetus are available. Classical CAH can be detected through newborn screening. CAH is treatable with medications. In its classical form, CAH requires lifelong medical management.

Children born with this disorder often experience an excess of androgen, which may lead to precocious puberty in boys and male characteristics and genital anomalies in females, with baby girls occasionally being misidentified as boys. Depending on the severity of the enzyme deficiency, congenital adrenal hyperplasia can remain undiagnosed for years. In severe cases, infants may experience dehydration, vomiting, and failure to thrive.

The nonclassical form of CAH (also known as late-onset or mild CAH) presents with milder symptoms, which may appear at any time from infancy through adulthood and is not characterized by ambiguous genitalia in girls. Instead, these individuals have a partial enzyme deficiency and therefore have better cortisol production, normal aldosterone production, and lower levels of adrenal androgens. The nonclassical form of CAH can result in rapid growth and premature puberty in early childhood, but some individuals may have shorter-than-expected height, hirsutism (excessive hair growth), irregular menstrual periods, acne, and more rarely, infertility in either males or females. In young women these features may be confused with polycystic ovary syndrome. Nonclassical CAH is not a life-threatening condition, but it can present serious quality-of-life issues for the individuals affected. Some people with nonclassical CAH are not symptomatic at all and are only identified because of an affected parent or sibling.

Overactive Adrenal Glands

The adrenal glands sometimes develop nodules that produce too much of certain hormones. Large nodules that exhibit particular features on imaging may be cancerous. Both benign and cancerous nodules can produce excessive amounts of certain hormones. When this occurs the condition is referred to as overactive adrenal glands. Symptoms and treatment depend on which hormones are being overproduced.

Hyperaldosteronism

Excess production of aldosterone from one or both adrenal glands is known as hyperaldosteronism. This disorder is characterized by an increase in blood pressure that may require a variety of medications to control. Some people with hyperaldosteronism can also develop low blood potassium levels, resulting in muscle aches, weakness, and spasms. When hyperaldosteronism is caused by a benign tumor in one adrenal gland, the disease is called Conn syndrome.

Pheochromocytoma

Pheochromocytoma is a rare, usually benign tumor that develops in one adrenal gland (although it can sometimes affect both glands) and results in bursts of excess adrenaline or noradrenaline from the adrenal medulla (see page 22). Occasionally neural crest tissue, which is similar to the adrenal medulla, may be the cause of overproduction of these hormones. This condition is called a paraganglioma.

Pheochromocytomas can cause persistent or episodic high blood pressure that may be difficult to control with regular medications. If left untreated, a pheochromocytoma can result in severe or life-threatening damage to other body systems, particularly the cardiovascular system. Additional symptoms include anxiety, headache, rapid heartbeat, sweating, and tremors. Most people with a pheochromocytoma are between the ages of twenty and fifty, but the tumor can emerge at any age; some people are genetically predisposed to developing it. Surgical removal of the pheochromocytoma usually returns blood pressure to normal.

Adrenal Cancer

Malignant adrenal tumors, such as adrenocortical carcinomas, are very rare. Certain genetic conditions may increase the risk for these tumors, which are typically fairly large, reaching several inches in diameter. Although this type of malignancy is potentially curable during the early stages, by the time the tumors are diagnosed, they usually have spread to distant organs and tissues (metastasized), most commonly the abdominal cavity, bone, liver, and lungs, and have caused numerous changes in the body from the excess hormones they produce. However, not all cancers found in adrenal glands began there; the majority are secondary cancers that started elsewhere in the body and spread to the adrenal glands.

Adrenal Insufficiency Symptoms and Diagnosis
SYMPTOMS OF ADRENAL INSUFFICIENCY

The signs and symptoms of adrenal insufficiency typically appear gradually over several months or longer. Because the symptoms progress slowly, they are often ignored until a stressful event, such as an accident or illness, causes them to become worse. The following are the most common symptoms of adrenal insufficiency:

- abdominal pain
- chronic or long-lasting fatigue
- loss of appetite
- muscle weakness
- weight loss

Additional symptoms may also include the following:

- amenorrhea (irregular or absent menstrual periods) in women
- depression
- diarrhea

- headache
- hypoglycemia (low blood sugar)
- hypotension (low blood pressure) that may cause dizziness and fainting upon standing
- irritability
- nausea
- salt cravings
- severe muscle or joint pains
- sexual disinterest or dysfunction in women
- sweating
- vomiting

Hyperpigmentation (darkening of the skin) can occur with Addison's disease but not with secondary adrenal insufficiency. The condition affects both exposed and nonexposed areas of the body and is visible primarily on the lips, mucous membranes, pressure points (such as the elbows, knees, knuckles, and toes), scars, and skin folds.

SYMPTOMS OF ADRENAL CRISIS

Sudden or severe worsening of adrenal insufficiency symptoms is called adrenal crisis. If the person has Addison's disease, it's known as an Addisonian crisis. Most people seek medical treatment before adrenal crisis occurs, but that isn't possible if the symptoms arise suddenly. Symptoms of adrenal crisis include the following:

- dehydration
- hyperkalemia (high blood potassium) and hyponatremia (low blood sodium)
- hypotension (low blood pressure)
- loss of consciousness
- severe vomiting and diarrhea
- sudden, severe pain in the abdomen, legs, or lower back

If untreated, adrenal crisis can be fatal. People with adrenal insufficiency who have weakness, nausea, or vomiting should seek immediate emergency treatment to prevent adrenal crisis and possible death. An injection of corticosteroid (a synthetic glucocorticoid hormone) can be lifesaving. Individuals with adrenal insufficiency should carry a corticosteroid injection with them at all times and ensure that their friends and family know how and when to administer it.

Diagnosing Adrenal Insufficiency

I t can be difficult to diagnose adrenal insufficiency, particularly in the early stages of the disease. It might only be suspected once a physician or other health-care provider reviews a patient's symptoms and medical history. Tests that measure the blood levels of cortisol and aldosterone are standard first steps. If levels are low, imaging studies of the adrenal and pituitary glands can help establish the cause and confirm a diagnosis.

HORMONAL BLOOD AND URINE TESTS

ACTH stimulation test. The ACTH stimulation test is the most common test used for diagnosing adrenal insufficiency. It measures how well the adrenal glands respond to adrenocorticotropic hormone (ACTH), the hormone produced in the pituitary gland that stimulates the adrenal glands to release cortisol (see page 20). During the test the patient is given an intravenous injection of synthetic ACTH, and samples of blood, urine, or both are taken before and after the injection. The cortisol levels in the blood and urine samples are then measured in a lab. Normal results for healthy individuals will show a rise in cortisol levels in the blood and urine after the ACTH injection. People who have Addison's disease, acute adrenal crisis, or long-standing secondary adrenal insufficiency will show little or no increase in cortisol levels. If secondary adrenal insufficiency has occurred very recently or is mild, the adrenal glands may still respond to ACTH because they haven't yet discontinued their own production of the hormone.

CRH stimulation test. When the response to the ACTH test is abnormal, a CRH stimulation test can help pinpoint the cause of adrenal insufficiency. A CRH stimulation test measures levels of cortisol in the blood before and after an intravenous injection of a synthetic form of corticotropin-releasing hormone (CRH). Blood samples are taken at four thirty-minute intervals after the injection and the cortisol levels are measured in a lab.

People with Addison's disease respond to this test by producing high levels of ACTH but no cortisol. People with secondary adrenal insufficiency will not produce ACTH, or their response will be delayed. A delayed ACTH response points to the hypothalamus as the cause. If the pituitary gland is damaged, CRH will not stimulate ACTH secretion, so a lack of ACTH response would point to the pituitary gland as the cause.

DIAGNOSING ADRENAL INSUFFICIENCY DURING ADRENAL CRISIS

A reliable diagnosis of adrenal insufficiency isn't possible when a person is in the midst of adrenal crisis. However, a measurement of blood ACTH and cortisol levels at the time of adrenal crisis, prior to treatment with corticosteroids, can help make a preliminary diagnosis. Low blood sodium, low blood glucose, and high blood potassium may also be present during the crisis. An ACTH stimulation test can be administered once the crisis is under control. If the diagnosis is still uncertain, additional lab tests may be necessary.

ADDITIONAL TESTING AFTER A DIAGNOSIS OF ADRENAL INSUFFICIENCY

Once a diagnosis of adrenal insufficiency has been confirmed, healthcare providers may order additional tests to help determine the cause of the insufficiency. Some of the various tests used can identify antibodies corresponding to autoimmune Addison's disease or verify whether the condition is associated with tuberculosis.

Abdominal ultrasound. An ultrasound scan—also called sonogram, diagnostic sonography, and ultrasonography—is administered by a specially trained technician who employs a device called a transducer, which uses high-frequency sound waves to create images of the inside of the body. These images can reveal abnormalities of the adrenal glands (such as a small size, an enlargement, nodules, or signs of calcium deposits) that could indicate bleeding.

Antibody blood tests. Antibodies are proteins made by the immune system to protect the body from foreign substances. In autoimmune disorders, the immune system mistakenly recognizes a natural body component as "foreign" and begins to attack healthy cells, causing the destruction of tissue. Antibody blood tests may be used for people diagnosed with adrenal insufficiency to identify antibodies associated with autoimmune Addison's disease.

Computerized tomography (CT) scan. A CT scan is a painless, commonly performed procedure that produces cross-sectional images of the body using X-rays and a computer. It can show the size and shape of the pituitary gland to determine if there is any abnormality. Prior to the procedure, the patient may receive an injection of a special dye called a contrast medium, which makes parts of the body show up more clearly in the image. For the scan, the patient lies on a table that slides into a large, tunnel-shaped device in which the X-rays are taken. CT scans are done in outpatient centers or hospitals. No anesthesia is needed. An X-ray technician performs the procedure, and a radiologist interprets the images.

Hormonal blood tests. Hormonal blood tests can evaluate how well the pituitary gland is functioning and gauge its ability to produce other hormones. Additional tests may be used by health-care providers to obtain a detailed view of the pituitary gland and assess how well it's functioning.

Magnetic resonance imaging (MRI). An MRI is a noninvasive medical procedure that uses a large magnet and radio waves to produce detailed pictures of the body's internal organs and soft tissues without using X-rays. MRIs can be used to produce a three-dimensional image of the hypothalamus and the pituitary gland to find out if an abnormality is present. A specially trained technician performs the procedure in an outpatient center or a hospital, and a radiologist interprets the images. An MRI may include the injection of contrast medium. During the scan, the patient lies on a table that slides inside a tunnel-shaped machine. The scan can take thirty to fifty minutes, and the patient must stay still during that entire time. As the MRI machine makes a lot of noise, the technician may offer the patient earplugs. Most MRI exams are painless and no anesthesia is needed. However, patients who find it difficult or uncomfortable to remain still during the MRI or who have claustrophobia (fear of closed-in spaces) may be given light sedation.

Tuberculin skin test. A tuberculin skin test involves putting some testing material, known as tuberculin, under the skin to measure how a patient's immune system reacts to the bacteria that cause tuberculosis (TB). The results can indicate whether the cause of the adrenal insufficiency could be related to TB. The test is done by a nurse or lab technician in a health-care provider's office. No anesthesia is needed. After two to three days, the patient returns to the provider's office so any reaction to the test can be evaluated.

A special blood test may also be used to determine whether the patient has a TB infection, which occurs when tuberculosis bacteria live in the body without causing illness. With tuberculosis disease, the TB bacteria actively attack the lungs and make the person ill. When that occurs, a chest X-ray and sputum sample may be required to make a positive diagnosis.

Treating Adrenal Insufficiency and Adrenal Crisis

HORMONE REPLACEMENT THERAPY

Adrenal insufficiency is treated by replacing the hormones the adrenal glands aren't making. The goal of treatment is to ensure proper hormone levels on a day-to-day basis, and most patients will require daily replacement hormones for the rest of their lives. Glucocorticoids (such as dexamethasone, hydrocortisone, or prednisone) will be needed to replace the cortisol the body is no longer manufacturing, and mineralocorticoids, called fludrocortisone acetate (Florinef), may be necessary for patients whose bodies aren't making aldosterone. People with secondary adrenal insufficiency generally maintain aldosterone production, so they don't require aldosterone replacement therapy.

During times of stress, such as with a serious illness or surgery, people with adrenal insufficiency may need extra glucocorticoids.

The dose of each medication must be customized by a physician to meet the unique needs of the individual patient.

Symptoms of adrenal crisis—such as low blood pressure, low blood glucose, low blood sodium, and high blood potassium—can be life-threatening. Standard emergency treatment involves immediate IV injections of corticosteroids and large volumes of an IV solution containing dextrose, a type of sugar. This intervention usually results in rapid improvement. If the patient can take liquids and medications by mouth, the amount of corticosteroids is decreased until a dose that maintains normal hormone levels is attained. If aldosterone is deficient, the patient will need to regularly take oral doses of fludrocortisone acetate.

COMPLICATIONS OF ADRENAL INSUFFICIENCY

Conditions that place added stress on the body—such as illness, severe injury, surgery, or pregnancy—can be especially difficult for people with adrenal insufficiency. Supplementary treatment may be necessary for them to recover and manage their health.

Illness

During an illness the patient's standard dose of oral corticosteroids may need to be increased to replicate the adrenal glands' normal response to stress. If the illness includes a high fever or severe injury, the dose may need to be doubled or even tripled. After recovery, dosing is gradually returned to the patient's normal (pre-illness) status. People with adrenal insufficiency should be instructed by their health-care providers how to appropriately increase their medication during such times of stress. Note that if severe diarrhea, infection, or vomiting occurs, immediate medical attention must be sought to avoid adrenal crisis.

Injury

Patients who experience a severe injury may need an increased dose of corticosteroids immediately following the injury as well as during recovery. Such "stress" doses are typically given intravenously. After recovery, the amount of corticosteroids is decreased to the patient's normal (preinjury) dose.

Pregnancy

The same hormone therapy a woman with adrenal insufficiency took prior to becoming pregnant will be continued during her pregnancy. However, if nausea or vomiting occurs early in the pregnancy and interferes with the patient's ability to take medication orally, it may be necessary to switch to injections of corticosteroids. Hormone treatment during delivery is similar to what is used during surgery (see below). After childbirth, the dose is gradually returned to the patient's normal (prepregnancy) dose.

Surgery

People with adrenal insufficiency who require any type of surgery that involves general anesthesia must be treated with intravenous (IV) corticosteroids and saline. The IV treatment will begin prior to surgery and continue until the patient is fully awake and able to take medication by mouth. The "stress" dose will be adjusted throughout the recovery period until the patient's normal (presurgery) dose is reached. People diagnosed with adrenal insufficiency who have taken long-term corticosteroids during the past year but who are not currently taking them should inform their health-care provider in advance of any surgery. Although they may have sufficient ACTH to carry them through the events of everyday life, they may need IV treatment to cope with the added stress of surgery.

NUTRITION AND ADRENAL INSUFFICIENCY

People with Addison's disease who are also deficient in aldosterone may benefit from following a sodium-rich diet. They should consult their health-care provider or a registered dietitian who can provide specific recommendations and appropriate food sources of sodium, along with daily sodium intake guidelines.

Because corticosteroid therapy is associated with an increased risk of osteoporosis—a medical condition in which the bones become less dense and more prone to fracture—people who take corticosteroids need to take extra precautions to protect the health of their bones. This includes consuming rich dietary sources of calcium and vitamin D (see page 123). Some people may also benefit from supplementation. A health-care provider or registered dietitian should be consulted to determine the appropriate type of supplement and dosage needed based on the individual's age and health.

TREATING AND PREVENTING ADRENAL CRISIS AND DEALING WITH EMERGENCIES

People with adrenal crisis need immediate treatment with adrenal hormones. Any delay in obtaining this treatment could result in death. If the person is vomiting or unconscious, the treatment must be injected instead of given orally. For this reason, individuals with adrenal insufficiency should always carry a corticosteroid injection and ensure that others around them know how and when to administer it.

If you have been diagnosed with adrenal insufficiency, follow these steps to prevent adrenal crisis or prepare for an emergency:

- If you are chronically weak or tired or are losing weight unintentionally, talk with your health-care provider about the possibility of adjusting the dose of your hormone therapy.
- Talk with your health-care provider about providing written instructions for how to increase your dose of corticosteroids when you're ill.
- Seek immediate emergency treatment if you suddenly become very ill, especially if you're vomiting and not able to take medication orally.
- Always carry identification and a card that states your condition as "adrenal insufficiency."
- Wear a medical-alert tag or bracelet that notifies emergency health-care providers of the need to inject corticosteroids should you become severely injured or incapacitated, or unconscious, or are unable to respond to questions.
- Always carry a needle, a syringe, and an injectable form of corticosteroids for emergencies.
- The medical-alert card or tag should also include the name and phone number of your health-care provider and the names and numbers of friends or family members to be notified in the event of an emergency.

3

C H A P T E R

*Great rationalizations.
All of which her adrenal gland
middle-fingered and then
carried right on.*

J. R. WARD
American novelist

"Adrenal Fatigue" Deconstructed

THE ADRENAL FATIGUE ENIGMA

drenal fatigue" is a constellation of diverse medical signs and symptoms, known as a syndrome, that is believed to result when the adrenal glands, along with the hypothalamus and pituitary gland, are functioning below their optimal levels as a result of chronic physical or emotional stress or the outcome of a lifetime of stress that takes a toll as we age. Over the past century, adrenal fatigue has gone by a variety of other names: adrenal apathy, adrenal burnout, adrenal exhaustion, adrenal neurasthenia, adrenal stress, non-Addison's hypoadrenia, neurasthenia, and subclinical hypoadrenia, among others. The concept of adrenal fatigue was conceived in 1998 by chiropractor and naturopath James Wilson, one of the founders of the Canadian College of Naturopathic Medicine in Toronto, Ontario. Since then his theories and approaches have become popularized among alternative health practitioners. However, the term is not recognized by any endocrinology society or medical group.

Theoretically, adrenal fatigue occurs when hormone levels drop, but unlike Addison's disease (see page 23), they don't drop low enough for current medical tests to detect an insufficiency. Consequently, laboratory results appear normal.

As explained in chapter two, the adrenal glands perform a variety of vital functions that are essential to life. These include, among others, controlling the body's response to stress, regulating blood pressure and heart rate, supporting the immune system, balancing the levels of salt and water in the body, and aiding the metabolism of carbo-hydrates, proteins, and fats. Proponents of adrenal fatigue syndrome believe that as we age or when we experience prolonged periods of stress—whether from work challenges, relationship problems, excessive physical exertion, repeated pregnancies, persistent infections, or chronic disease—the adrenal glands begin to weaken, just like other parts of the body over time. Eventually the adrenals may become incapable of responding adequately when they're needed.

People diagnosed with "adrenal fatigue" typically exhibit a spectrum of symptoms, such as low energy levels, a reduced ability to handle stress, and a weakened immune system. They usually report feeling constantly tired and unrefreshed, even after many hours of sleep. Consequently, they may resort to stimulants, such as caffeinated beverages, energy shots, or sugary foods, just to make it through the day.

Clinical adrenal dysfunction isn't acknowledged by conventional medicine until the adrenal glands virtually stop working and the condition becomes life-threatening (Addison's disease). With purported adrenal fatigue, however, the speculation is that the adrenals and related organs are still doing their jobs, but their performance levels are subpar. Although the results of standard medical tests may show hormone levels in the "normal" range, the patient is suffering nonetheless.

The HPA Axis

Although the term "stress" rightfully carries many negative connotations, it describes an important neurobehavioral and physiological response that is intrinsic to life. When confronted with an environmental stressor, the body quickly orchestrates changes in brain activity that are followed shortly thereafter by the secretion of what are called stress mediators, which include cytokines, metabolic hormones, and corticosteroids. These circulating chemical messages then act in the brain and on peripheral tissues to modify physiological processes and behavioral effects. The primary pathway that regulates our stress response is known as the hypothalamic-pituitary-adrenal (HPA) axis. The stress response coordinated by the HPA axis is a well-choreographed, multisystem response involving behavioral, physiological, and metabolic actions, with tightly regulated components that must be activated at the right times and in the right contexts.

Normal functioning of the HPA axis ensures that the body responds appropriately to altered environmental demands, equipping it with an essential system to promote survival. Stress activates the HPA axis, initiating a cascade of neuroendocrine (both neural and endocrine in structure or function) signals that trigger the release of hormones and neurotransmitters, such as cortisol, epinephrine (adrenaline), and norepinephrine (noradrenaline). Persistent activation of the stress-response system can, over time, undermine the ability of cells, tissues, and organ systems to rapidly respond to changes in physiological need and can compromise the long-term capability of the body to respond to these changes.

To understand the theories behind adrenal fatigue, it's essential to also understand what the three organs of the HPA axis do and how they interact. When these organs aren't functioning at their peak, the condition is known as HPA axis dysfunction or dysregulation (HPA-D). Both adrenal dysfunction and HPA-D denote the same condition, and the terms are often used interchangeably. However, HPA-D is a

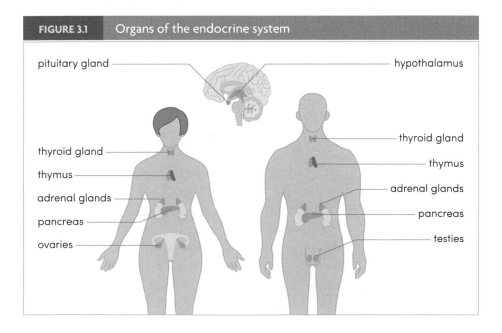

FIGURE 3.1   Organs of the endocrine system

pituitary gland ———————————   ——————— hypothalamus

                                                              ——————— thyroid gland
thyroid gland ———————   ——————— thymus
thymus ———————   ——————— adrenal glands
adrenal glands ———————   ——————— pancreas
pancreas ———————   ——————— testies
ovaries ———————

more accurate description of what is actually happening physiologically, and therefore it's a more medically accepted choice.

When we experience any type or level of stress, the hypothalamus (see below) releases corticotropin-releasing hormone (CRH). The release of CRH sends a signal to the pituitary gland to release another hormone, adrenocorticotropic hormone (ACTH). After its release, ACTH travels through the bloodstream to the adrenal glands, where it triggers the release of cortisol, a steroid hormone. Cortisol prepares the body for the fight-or-flight response by flooding it with glucose to create a burst of energy while simultaneously suppressing the digestive system, the production of insulin, the immune response, and the reproductive system, so all energy is directed toward fighting or fleeing.

The HPA axis is essentially a messaging loop: the output of one of the glands loops around and becomes input for another gland in the axis. In healthy individuals, when the receptors in the hypothalamus and pituitary gland receive signals from the adrenal glands that high levels of cortisol have been released, they stop production of CRH and ACTH, which then triggers the adrenals to reduce their production of cortisol. These processes are known as negative feedback loops. When cortisol levels have decreased, the stress response concludes, the body relaxes, and hormone levels stabilize. As we age, the hypothalamus and pituitary gland become less sensitive to negative feedback from cortisol (that is, they become less able to quickly terminate the stress response), and both ACTH and cortisol levels rise. Interestingly, young women produce lower levels of cortisol in response to stress than do young men, and older women secrete more cortisol in response to stress than do older men.

HYPOTHALAMUS

The word "hypothalamus" comes from two Greek words that translate to "under thalamus," which correlates to the exact location of the hypothalamus in the brain: underneath the thalamus (see page 128) and above the pituitary gland (see page 45). Although the hypothalamus comprises a small area of the brain, it has a large and important job influencing both the endocrine and nervous systems.

The primary function of the hypothalamus is to keep the body's systems in balance, a state known as homeostasis. As such, it has a vital role in many body functions, including regulating the following:

- appetite
- blood pressure
- body fluids
- body temperature
- childbirth
- electrolyte balance
- emotions
- heart rate
- production of digestive juices
- sex drive
- sleep cycles
- thirst
- weight

When any of the body's systems are out of balance, the affected areas send signals to the brain to alert the hypothalamus. In turn, the hypothalamus responds by releasing the necessary hormones into the bloodstream to bring the system back into homeostasis. For example, the body maintains an internal temperature of about 98.6 degrees F. If the hypothalamus receives a signal that the body is too hot, it will instruct the body to perspire. If it receives a signal that the body's temperature has dropped too low, it will instruct the body to create more heat by shivering.

To regulate the body's systems, the hypothalamus creates or controls many of the hormones in the body. It also works closely with the pituitary gland, which creates and releases other essential hormones. These two organs work together to manage the endocrine system, which includes the adrenal glands, kidneys, and thyroid gland.

The hypothalamus produces and secretes seven different hormones:

Antidiuretic hormones (ADH), also called arginine vasopressin, tells the kidneys how much water to conserve. It constantly regulates and balances the amount of water in the blood, which affects both blood volume and blood pressure, and controls the concentration of urine excreted by the kidneys.

Corticotropin-releasing hormone (CRH), also known as corticotropin-releasing factor or corticoliberin, controls the body's response to physical and emotional stress. It helps regulate metabolism and immune response by coordinating with the pituitary and adrenal glands to release certain steroids.

Gonadotropin-releasing hormone (GnRH) stimulates the release of hormones connected to the sex organs and is important to reproductive function, puberty, and sexual maturation.

Growth hormone-releasing hormone (GHRH) controls growth and physical development in children and regulates metabolism in adults.

Oxytocin is a powerful hormone that acts as a neurotransmitter in the brain. It helps regulate a wide range of body processes and is greatly stimulated during sex, birth, and breastfeeding. It also plays roles in human behavior and psychology, including maternal-infant bonding, empathy, generosity, social interactions, trust, and orgasm. When we hug or kiss a loved one, oxytocin levels rise, which inspired its nicknames "love hormone," "hug hormone," and "cuddle hormone."

Somatostatin is a hormone that affects several areas of the body by inhibiting the secretion of other hormones, such as somatotropin (growth hormone), insulin (essential for the metabolism of carbohydrates and the regulation of glucose levels in the blood), and gastrin (a hormone that stimulates the secretion of gastric juice and is secreted into the bloodstream by the stomach wall in response to the presence of food).

Thyrotropin-releasing hormone (TRH) stimulates production of the thyroid hormone, which in turn controls brain development, the cardiovascular system, digestive health, energy levels, metabolism, and muscle control.

Because the hypothalamus plays such a critical role in the body, it's important to keep it healthy. The hypothalamus regulates appetite, but it's also affected by foods that are eaten. Studies confirm that diets high in saturated fats, particularly those from animal-based foods (meat and dairy products), can alter the processes of the hypothalamus that regulate hunger and energy. They also have an inflammatory effect on the body. This can negatively influence the immune system and increase inflammation in the digestive tract.

PITUITARY GLAND

The pituitary, also called the hypophysis and the "master gland," is a pea-sized gland that sits in the small, bony cavity at the base of the brain. It produces several different hormones that travel throughout the body managing certain functions and stimulating other glands to produce other hormones.

The following hormones are created in the anterior (front part) of the pituitary gland:

Adrenocorticotropic hormone (ACTH), also called corticotropin or adrenocorticotropin, stimulates the production of cortisol by the adrenal glands. Cortisol is important in controlling metabolism, blood sugar levels, and blood pressure. It's also an anti-inflammatory and is produced in larger amounts during times of stress, illness, or injury.

FIGURE 3.2	Hormones of the endocrine system

Hypothalamus
TRH, CRH, GHRH
Dopamine
Somatostatin
Vasopressin

Thyroid and Parathyroid
T3, T4
Calcitonin
PTH

Liver
IGF, THPO

Adrenal
Androgens
Glucocorticoids
Adrenaline
Noradrenaline

Kidney
Calcitrol
Renin
Erythropoietin

Testes
Androgens
Estradiol
Inhibin

Pineal gland
Melatonin

Pituitary Gland
GH, TSH, ACTH, FSH, MSH, LH
Prolactin
Oxytocin
Vasopressin

Thymus
Thymopoietin

Stomach
Gastrin
Ghrelin
Histamine
Somatostatin
Neuropeptide Y

Pancreas
Insulin
Glucagon
Somatostatin

Ovary, Placenta
Estrogens
Progesterone

Uterus
Prolactin
Relaxin

Follicle-stimulating hormone (FSH) in women stimulates the ovaries to produce estrogen and develop eggs and in men promotes sperm production. Luteinizing hormone (see below) and FSH work together to enable normal function of the ovaries and testes.

Growth hormone (GH), also called somatotropin or human growth hormone, is synthesized and secreted by anterior pituitary cells called somatotrophs. GH stimulates growth in childhood and is important for maintaining bone mass, muscle mass, and fat distribution in adults. It also promotes healing and supports immune system health.

Luteinizing hormone (LH) stimulates the production of testosterone in men and ovulation (egg release) in women.

Prolactin works with other hormones to stimulate the production of breast milk after childbirth. It also affects sex hormone levels and fertility in both women and men.

Thyroid-stimulating hormone (TSH) stimulates the thyroid gland to produce thyroid hormones, which regulate the body's energy balance, growth, metabolism, and nervous system activity.

The posterior (back part) of the pituitary gland does not produce hormones but rather stores and secretes hormones produced by the hypothalamus. The following hormones are stored in the posterior pituitary:

Antidiuretic hormone (see page 43).

Oxytocin (see page 44).

HPA Axis Dysfunction
ALLOSTATIC LOAD

Allostasis, which literally means "maintaining stability," is the process by which the body's state of internal, physiological balance (homeostasis) is maintained in response to actual or perceived environmental and psychological stressors. The body responds to stress with self-regulating, allostatic processes aimed at returning critical systems to a set point within a narrow range of operation that ensures the body's survival. These self-regulating processes include multiple behavioral and physiological components.

Over the past several decades, increasing evidence supports the hypothesis that disruption of the HPA axis can lead to a dysregulated stress response, exacting a physiological toll commonly referred to as allostatic load. The concept of allostatic load was proposed to refer to the wear and tear the body experiences due to repeated cycles of allostasis, as well as to the inefficient turning on and shutting off of these responses. Researchers have acknowledged that a high allostatic load can contribute to increased health vulnerabilities and inappropriate responses to stressors that might underlie abnormal coping strategies and many neuropsychiatric disorders, such as anxiety and depression.

The stress response is an essential brain–body reaction that protects homeostasis and ensures survival in the face of threatening environmental stimuli. This coordinated response that follows a stressful situation allows mediators of allostasis to mobilize, letting the body adapt to a temporary environmental shift. As such, healthy allostatic responses are protective and a sign of resilience. However, if allostatic mediators are overactive, improperly regulated, poorly terminated, or engaged inappropriately, the allostatic burden can increase. Eventually this results in allostatic overload, which, rather than protecting the body, leads to a stream of failures in multiple physiological systems. Consequently, the systems that usually impart resilience result instead in increased vulnerability.

Given the central role of the HPA axis stress response in allostatic processes, it's not surprising that disruptions in the biological reaction to stress can lead to changes in nerve impulse function, behavior, and immune function, and also contribute to negative physical and mental health outcomes. In fact, disruption of normal HPA function is a hallmark of a varied set of physical and neuropsychiatric diseases, including anxiety disorders, depression, post-traumatic stress disorder (PTSD), and metabolic dysfunction. These conditions affect millions of people worldwide, saddling them with significant economic and personal burdens. Whether these changes in HPA activity are a cause or consequence of such disease states is currently unclear, but it's reasonable to speculate that disrupting the normal self-regulating responses to environmental stress will predispose individuals to detrimental health consequences.

To protect against prolonged hormonal activity, the HPA axis is carefully modulated through negative feedback loops (see page 42) designed to maintain predetermined hormone levels (set points) and homeostasis. These delicately balanced negative feedback mechanisms keep the secretion of ACTH and cortisol within a comparatively narrow range. This function is exceedingly important, because too much or too little exposure to cortisol can have adverse consequences to overall health and result in serious harm to the body.

When a person experiences prolonged chronic stress, the normal release of hormones via the HPA axis is accelerated. In time, the overproduction of these hormones desensitizes the affiliated glands of the HPA axis, and they no longer recognize the signals to stop producing hormones. In other words, the negative feedback loop ceases to work as it should and HPA axis dysfunction becomes habituated.

In recent years the notion of adrenal fatigue has been popularized in natural and alternative health circles. Although many alternative practitioners are focusing on the adrenal glands being fatigued as a result of chronic stress, that is only one possible piece of the puzzle. More likely, if such a syndrome exists, it is the potential dysfunction of the entire HPA axis and its feedback loops that are causing symptoms, not merely a dysfunction in the adrenal glands.

FACTORS THAT INFLUENCE HPA AXIS HEALTH

A healthy stress response is characterized by a quick rise in cortisol levels, followed by a rapid decline after the termination of the stressful event. When the body is burdened by cumulative stress, however, the cortisol load increases. This results in wear and tear on cells, tissues, and organs from excessive exposure to the destructive properties of glucocorticoids, stress peptides, and proinflammatory cytokines. Because this load taxes the health of the individual and can influence the development of neuropsychiatric and metabolic disorders, it is essential to understand the systems that regulate cortisol production.

Three main determinants of HPA axis activity control the amount of cortisol a person is exposed to during adulthood: genetic history, early life events, and current life stressors. In addition, studies have found that PTSD can also contribute to HPA axis disturbances.

Genetic factors. Differences among individuals in cortisol responses to stress result from a complex interplay between genetic and environmental factors. The genetic contribution to the variability in HPA axis reactivity is believed to arise from DNA variations in the genes encoding the neurotransmitters involved in HPA axis regulation.

Early life influences. Prenatal stress may activate the release of stress hormones, such as glucocorticoids, that play important roles in the development of fetal immune organs and immune cells. Perinatal stress sets the stage for subsequent disease and can have a powerful influence on health. These early stressors are independent risk factors and are distinctly different from other factors, such as genetic susceptibility or lifestyle influences in later life. Studies show that pre- and postnatal processes contribute to the lifelong responsiveness of the HPA axis to stressors. For example, prenatal alcohol exposure is associated with impaired HPA axis responsiveness in adulthood. Maternal stress during gestation also modifies the HPA axis responsivity in both infant and adult offspring.

Recent studies have focused on the consequences of early childhood events on the stress response. Childhood trauma is associated with mental and physical health problems in adulthood, as well as with alterations in HPA axis function. Hypotheses suggest that exposure to sexual, emotional, and physical abuse during critical periods of brain development in childhood may permanently alter stress responsivity. This alteration in stress responsivity may explain why exposure to adverse events during childhood is a risk factor for the development of alcohol and other drug abuse problems in adulthood, as well as for anxiety and depressive disorders.

Current life stressors. Periods of severe, ongoing stress in adulthood, such as chronic illness, family problems, job pressures, neighborhood violence, exposure to combat, or the development of neuropsychiatric disorders, alter the HPA axis dynamic and increase the cortisol burden, independent of the influence of prenatal and childhood stressors. Chronic stress triggers an allostatic shift in the normal circadian rhythm of cortisol release, as well as in stress-induced cortisol levels. Consequently, after chronic stress baseline cortisol levels rise, the body's cortisol response to acute stress is diminished, so it takes longer for cortisol levels elevated by high stress to return to normal (prestress) levels. Each compromise to allostasis makes the HPA axis more sensitive, resulting in increased cortisol exposure and a greater cortisol burden following each stressful episode.

Post-traumatic stress disorder (PTSD). The HPA axis has been a primary focus of neuroendocrine research in PTSD. Studies show that people with PTSD have lower afternoon levels of cortisol than control subjects, and women with PTSD have significantly lower cortisol levels than women without PTSD. The specific type of trauma experienced by a person also makes a difference. For example, cortisol levels are significantly lower in people who have experienced physical or sexual abuse. These findings highlight the complexity of the relationship between HPA axis activity and PTSD pathophysiology. Regardless of whether underlying HPA axis dysfunction precedes PTSD symptoms, evidence suggests that dysregulation occurs through an increased sensitivity of the negative feedback mechanisms that regulate the HPA axis, and this results in lower levels of circulating cortisol.

Adrenal Fatigue and the Disease Continuum

Supporters of the concept of adrenal fatigue believe the syndrome could be affecting millions of people worldwide. However, adrenal fatigue isn't currently an accepted medical diagnosis. It's both interesting and somewhat alarming that such a potentially widespread dysfunction has been castigated by brilliant contemporary physicians around the globe and yet has generated so much interest among the public. Why is there such a wide-scale disconnect?

The basis for conventional medicine rejecting or questioning the existence of adrenal fatigue is multilayered:

1. Is there evidence that chronic, acute, or prolonged stress can lead to an imbalance or suboptimal levels of adrenal hormones?

2. Can that reduced hormonal output be quantified?

3. Can the quantifiable imbalance (if it exists) be proven to be the cause of the reported symptoms?

Neuroscientific research has demonstrated that stress, whether physical or emotional, is a powerful trigger for the release of adrenal hormones, such as adrenaline and cortisol. For example, during times of acute stress, adrenaline levels rapidly rise, and during times of rest, they gradually drop. Although we know that hormone levels are affected by stress, the degree to which these levels rise and fall varies greatly from person to person, and in some people these fluctuations may be barely noticeable. Also, when stress is chronic, these types of acute hormonal shifts don't occur. It's not surprising that laboratory measurements of "stress hormones" differ widely depending on the individual, the circumstances, and the type and level of stress experienced. So while it's clear that stress contributes to hormone imbalance in various ways, subclinical levels can't yet be accurately quantified and therefore don't meet the threshold for what conventional medicine considers scientific evidence.

Do subclinical hormone imbalances lead to clinical symptoms of fatigue? Because of the enormous variances among individuals, it's possible that some people could have clinically abnormal adrenaline output yet not feel fatigued, while other people may feel exhausted but their adrenaline levels are in the normal range. At this time there are no quantitative tests that can accurately show a conclusive connection between particular levels of any single adrenal hormone and symptoms of fatigue.

On the one hand, because current laboratory tests don't have the capacity to measure subclinical states, these tests may not realistically be useful for diagnosing adrenal fatigue. On the other hand, it's possible the current tests have value but the reference ranges need to be readjusted or the thresholds lowered to accurately reflect subclinical states.

We know conclusively that many degenerative diseases and common causes of death, including heart disease and cancer, can take several years or even decades to develop before symptoms are clinically detectable. However, our current laboratory tests and clinical detection methods lack the sensitivity to identify the signs of early disease. Although a person may appear outwardly healthy, genetic predisposition or a lifetime of poor nutrition, stress, and exposure to environmental contaminants may be taking an imperceptible toll.

It's not unusual for a person to feel seriously ill yet appear to be symptom-free and have normal laboratory test results. Conventional

Adrenal Fatigue or HPA Axis Dysfunction?

When we strive to understand and describe complicated medical conditions, it's tempting to minimize their complexity with simple names and explanations. Although doing this may initially help patients and the public make sense of perplexing disorders, it ultimately downplays the important mechanisms related to chronic conditions and can hinder the exploration of beneficial treatments and solutions. The use of the terms "adrenal fatigue" and "adrenal exhaustion" to encapsulate the complex dysfunction of the stress response is an example of this. While these terms have helped quash the notion that only extreme dysfunction of the adrenal glands—such as Addison's disease, adrenal crisis, or Cushing's disease—are worthy of clinical acknowledgment and investigation, many complementary and alternative health practitioners have begun suggesting that they be replaced with more medically precise terms, such as "HPA axis dysfunction."

Common laboratory testing methods assess the function of the HPA axis by measuring hormones secreted by the adrenal glands, primarily cortisol and dehydroepiandrosterone (DHEA). However, the mechanisms that control these hormone levels are, for the most part, separate from the adrenals. Cortisol production is governed primarily by the brain, central nervous system, and tissue-specific regulatory mechanisms, not the adrenal glands themselves. So although low cortisol and DHEA may be related to chronic stress, when levels drop as a result of HPA axis adaptation to protect the body from excess cortisol, the process has little to do with the capability of the adrenal glands to produce these hormones. The vast majority of people with low cortisol levels have normally functioning adrenal glands; their problem originates in the brain and central nervous system.

Using descriptive, medically appropriate terminology helps health-care providers and patients better understand the pathophysiology caused by stress and the stress medicine generally refrains from labeling a person as ill until the threshold for what's considered normal in terms of laboratory value references is crossed. These value references are derived from data based on the general population, and for that reason they don't and can't incorporate or reflect the broad range of individual variances.

So while modern testing methods are tremendously valuable for diagnosing catastrophic illness, they presently are incapable of detecting subclinical progressive disease states, such as borderline

response system. Why is the nomenclature important? In most situations, conditions related to perceived stress and its effects will have more to do with a treatment protocol that modulates the HPA axis and related glucocorticoid signaling than one that solely influences the adrenal glands. For example, many adaptogenic herbs and nutrients that were once thought to primarily support adrenal function have shown to actually have mechanisms that help regulate non-adrenal HPA axis functions.

The term "adrenal fatigue" is virtually absent from the vast amount of peer-reviewed literature that describes patient outcomes related to stress and HPA axis function. Additionally, there has been a push in the medical community to warn the public against the diagnostic "myth" of adrenal fatigue and to be suspicious of any health practitioners who use this term.

An expanding body of scientific research has linked a variety of chronic dysfunctions with specific patterns of adrenal hormone output. Therefore, using more medically descriptive terms not only enhances greater understanding of this important phenomenon, but it also encourages the development of appropriate therapies that address the complexity and interconnectedness of the entire stress response system. More appropriate terms would be "HPA axis dysfunction," "HPA axis dysregulation," and "stress maladaptation," as these connect stress with a host of measurable negative results related to the stress response that can be linked to processes regulated by the HPA axis. It's likely that these or similar terms will eventually replace "adrenal fatigue" and other surrogate descriptions for stress-related disorders, helping to dispel the belief that only life-threatening issues related to adrenal function are of clinical significance.

adrenal dysfunction and borderline hormonal, metabolic, or electro-lyte imbalances. The current medical framework defines "normal" as the absence of any detectable illness exhibited by laboratory test results that fall within a statistical range based on mathematical averages. Therefore, if lab results don't reflect the minimum stan-dardized levels for suboptimal function, the patient will be deemed healthy, despite contrary symptomatology. In other words, a person is considered either healthy or sick—there's no continuum or in-between stage.

If there's no demonstrable pathology to define disease, then according to conventional medicine, disease is nonexistent. But because the threshold for what is considered normal or abnormal is based on averages, not individuals, using laboratory testing as the sole definitive diagnostic tool is inherently flawed. Many peo-ple who have normal test results may be ill, but they're told that nothing is wrong with them and they're ushered out of the doctor's office and sent home. However, by the time laboratory tests detect a problem, the illness may have advanced too far to be treatable. Both scenarios do patients a disservice and cause needless suffering. Every untreated chronic or serious illness, from cancer to diabetes to hypertension, progresses from normal to severe over time, so it's only common sense that mild dysfunction of the adrenal glands or HPA axis exists, regardless of what it's called.

Without knowing the cause of illness, any treatment must be considered a guess.

RICHARD DIAZ, American author and fitness coach

Conventional medicine has dismissed claims of adrenal fatigue in much the same way it once rejected claims of other syndromes, such as chronic fatigue syndrome (CFS), fibromyalgia, premen-strual syndrome (PMS), Raynaud's syndrome, and irritable bowel syndrome (IBS), for which no standardized medical tests currently exist. Although mainstream physicians don't refute the symptoms of "adrenal fatigue" as reported by sufferers, they believe the root cause lies outside the adrenal glands and is more likely attributable to depression, CFS, or fibromyalgia than adrenal issues. What's fascinating is that not all that long ago, conventional medicine considered these very same diagnoses baseless!

Contrarily, practitioners of natural and alternative medicine, including naturopathic physicians and practitioners of functional, integrative, and traditional Chinese medicine, acknowledge the existence of adrenal fatigue syndrome and offer treatments for it. However, conventional physicians argue that accepting a medically unrecognized diagnosis from an "unqualified" health-care practitioner and using unproven remedies could make a patient feel worse because the true underlying cause of the symptoms remains undiagnosed and untreated. Bearing in mind the turnabout of the medical establishment with regard to other syndromes it once considered invalid but has now come to recognize, study, and even treat, would it be prudent to similarly embrace the possibility that adrenal fatigue syndrome is real?

Perhaps. But that approach is also a common and clever strategy for creating lucrative "fake" diseases, because knowing where to draw the line between what is healthy and unhealthy is a genuine medical quandary. It's easy for unscrupulous practitioners to take a true medical condition (such as adrenal insufficiency) and claim that a milder version of it (i.e., adrenal fatigue) also constitutes a real disease. For example, doctors have long debated where to draw the line between normal blood pressure and hypertension. The line keeps moving, and that's a legitimate medical controversy. Probably the best way to resolve these concerns is to conduct clinical studies to determine who benefits from treatment: the patient or the practitioner.

4

Until you have stood
in another woman's stilettos,
you will never begin to know
the year of pain she felt
breaking them in.

SHANNON L. ALDER
American author

The Progression
of "Adrenal Fatigue"

T he condition referred to as adrenal fatigue syndrome (AFS) is associated with a myriad of signs and symptoms, and each of these symptoms conceivably can be connected to a possible deficiency in one or more of the hormones produced by the HPA axis. Currently there is no definitive laboratory test to confirm or disconfirm a diagnosis of AFS, but if a person is suffering from a high number of these symptoms, champions of AFS would say it points to "adrenal fatigue" as the likely cause.

Ideally cortisol levels fluctuate according to circadian cycles, peaking in the morning and decreasing incrementally to a low at bedtime, only to rise again overnight. Among the hallmarks of purported adrenal fatigue are cortisol levels that are too high at night and not high enough in the morning. Alternative health practitioners contend that one reason standard blood tests are unable to detect these irregularities is because the tests are performed at whatever time is convenient for the doctor or laboratory, whereas a more effective diagnostic approach would be to test hormone levels at various times of the day, as doing so is far more likely to reveal an abnormal pattern of cortisol or DHEA secretion.

Unlike adrenal insufficiency and adrenal crisis, adrenal fatigue syndrome, if it exists, isn't life-threatening. However, because the causes of these conditions and the presumed cause of "adrenal fatigue" are similar (reduced or erratic secretion of adrenal hormones), it's not surprising that many symptoms of alleged adrenal fatigue parallel those of adrenal insufficiency. The most common symptoms associated with AFS include the following:

- alternating diarrhea and constipation
- anxiety
- body aches
- changes in appetite
- cravings for salty foods
- decreased ability to handle stress
- depression
- difficulty getting out of bed in the morning
- difficulty recovering from infections
- digestive problems; gastritis
- disinterest in sex; low sex drive
- dry skin
- fatigue that's unrelieved by sleep
- heart palpitations
- high incidence of flu and other respiratory illnesses
- higher energy levels in the evenings
- hypoglycemia (low blood sugar)
- insomnia; inability to fall asleep despite being tired
- joint pain
- lethargy
- low body temperature
- memory problems
- mood disorders
- multiple food and/or environmental allergies
- muscle weakness
- overuse of stimulants, such as caffeine and sugar
- panic attacks

- premature menopause in women
- rage attacks
- recurrent infections
- sleep disturbances
- thinning of the skin
- trouble thinking clearly (brain fog)
- unexplained hair loss
- unexplained pain in upper back or neck
- worsening PMS symptoms in women

Note that many health conditions and the drugs used to treat them can increase a person's risk of adrenal insufficiency. In addition, actual adrenal imbalance can be a component of a wide range of medical conditions, many of which may seem unrelated. These may include the following (among others):

- arthritis
- cancer
- chronic fatigue syndrome (CFS)
- diabetes mellitus
- fibromyalgia
- heart disease
- hypertension (high blood pressure)
- hypotension (low blood pressure)
- hypothyroidism (underactive thyroid gland)
- inflammatory bowel disease (Crohn's disease and ulcerative colitis)
- Lyme disease
- pernicious anemia

Potential Causes of "Adrenal Fatigue"

The purpose of the adrenal glands is to adapt the body to stressors. A natural cycle of stress, adaptation, and recovery allows the body to acclimate to environmental changes and stimuli and grow stronger through the process. However, when stressors override our ability to adapt effectively, or if the stress response is chronic, the body's vital reserves become depleted, impeding the body's ability to heal itself.

Excessive stress can arise from a variety of diverse sources. Contributing to our physical burden of stress are addictions (drug or alcohol), chemical exposure, chronic illness, disease, injury, overuse of drugs (pharmaceuticals, illicit drugs, over-the-counter medications), pollution, recurrent infections, and surgery. But stress may also be due to psychological or emotional factors, including the daily demands of modern life, mental illness or mental health problems, work difficulties, worry, and a host of chronic health and lifestyle factors, including the following:

- abuse (physical, sexual, emotional)
- autoimmune disorders
- blood sugar imbalances
- cigarette smoking
- electrolyte imbalances
- excessive consumption of sugary or highly refined foods
- food sensitivities
- frequent exposure to environmental toxins
- frequent infections (bacterial, viral, yeast)
- intestinal inflammation
- lack of sleep
- nutritional deficiencies
- overconsumption of alcohol
- overweight or obesity
- persistent mental or emotional stress
- physical trauma or injury
- poor dietary habits, skipping meals, eating irregularly

CHRONIC INFECTIONS

Chronic infections can be located anywhere in the body, although they often originate in infected teeth or gums. Infections cause inflammation and stress that trigger the inflammatory response and the release of adrenal hormones, such as cortisol. Intestinal infections also give rise to the inflammatory response, but these may occur subclinically, with no obvious signs. Common intestinal infections include fungal dysbiosis, giardia, *Helicobacter pylori* (*H. pylori*), and small intestinal bacterial overgrowth (SIBO), among others.

I've been sick for so long, I don't remember a time when I wasn't.

DALISON G. BAILEY, *Present Perfect*

ENVIRONMENTAL TOXINS

Every day we are exposed to thousands of chemicals in our air, water, and food. From personal-care products to toothpaste and dental fillings, and from cleaning products to carpeting, clothing, and furniture, chemicals enter our environment and bodies (through air, food, skin, and water) on a regular and unavoidable basis, further adding to the body's toxic load. Additional environmental stressors, particularly in urban areas, are noise pollution and electromagnetic exposure from cell phones, microwave towers, and appliances, such as computers, wearable electronics, and microwave ovens.

NUTRITIONAL DEFICIENCIES

When we're under stress, our nutrient needs are greater than usual. A diet low in micronutrients, plant foods, and fiber but high in refined carbohydrates, low-quality fats, and sugar adds to the body's stress burden and makes it difficult for the body's systems to function properly. Lack of hydration and contaminated water affect electrolyte balance. And poor eating habits, such as not eating meals at regular times, eating on the run, and relying on fast food and animal protein (meat, eggs, and dairy), contribute not only to nutrient deficiencies but also to inadequate digestion. In addition, food sensitivities can damage the intestines and inhibit the absorption of nutrients. Internally, toxins may be generated due to microbial imbalances in the gut and impaired digestion. When food is not properly digested, it may ferment in the intestines, producing harmful substances that can be absorbed through the intestinal lining. As the body's toxic load increases, its inherent ability to eliminate toxins decreases, creating a vicious cycle of ongoing physical stress.

STIMULANTS AND EXCESSIVE EXERCISE

Although we normally think of stimulants in the form of drugs (pharmaceutical, over-the-counter, and recreational), there are many socially acceptable forms of stimulants that people consume on a regular basis, such as alcohol, caffeine, chocolate, and sugar. But other environmental stimulants are also pervasive in our contemporary world: loud music and noise, upsetting current events, tragic news, and violence. Even fear-inducing or suspenseful movies and books can stimulate our adrenals to shift into overdrive by propelling our emotions into fight-or-flight mode. Less obvious but equally important stimulants include anger, fear, and rage, as well as "happy" emotions, such as anticipation, excitement, and infatuation. High-risk or extreme sports and excessive exercise can provide a temporary though compelling "high," in part by activating the secretion of higher-than-normal amounts of adrenal hormones.

Stages of "Adrenal Fatigue"

Alternative health practitioners have identified four stages that they believe "adrenal fatigue" progresses through, with advancing severity at each stage. Although what's been described as adrenal fatigue is not currently recognized by the mainstream medical community, this index may be helpful for diagnosing or treating patients at various levels of adrenal distress, as it paints a broad picture of what might be presented clinically. These stages somewhat parallel but expand upon Hans Selye's GAS model (see page 5). According to supporters of adrenal fatigue, the progression of the condition can vary significantly from person to person and is dependent on a wide variety of factors. Note that these stages are theoretical, not substantiated.

STAGE 1: ALARM REACTION

During this stage the body mounts an aggressive response to a stressor, mediated by an increase in antistress hormones, such as cortisol and dehydroepiandrosterone (DHEA). The needed amount of these hormones remains within normal levels, and the adrenal glands are able to handle the stress being placed on the body. Hormone production may be slightly affected, but for the most part the body is able to produce enough cortisol and DHEA to compensate. Fatigue is generally quite mild and usually occurs in the morning upon awakening or in midafternoon. No physical or physiological dysfunction is clinically observable. Normal daily function is expected, although peak performance isn't achievable. To counteract fatigue, people may turn to coffee, caffeinated sodas, energy shots, chocolate, or sugary, high-carbohydrate foods. These compensatory actions are generally socially acceptable and may even be considered a "normal" part of modern living.

STAGE 2: RESISTANCE RESPONSE

When the body is under constant or severe stress, cortisol levels continue to rise and DHEA levels start to gradually decrease. The adrenal cortex (see page 20) produces corticosteroids for this resistance response. Although normal daily activities can still be carried out, fatigue is more pronounced by the end of each day and the body requires more rest than usual to recover. As the stress-response system becomes overwhelmed, the adrenals begin to struggle, and symptoms such as body aches, depression, digestive problems, disrupted sleep patterns, elevated blood pressure, heart palpitations, hyperventilation, irritability, jitteriness, loss of appetite, menstrual irregularities, nervousness, weight gain, and a sensation of feeling

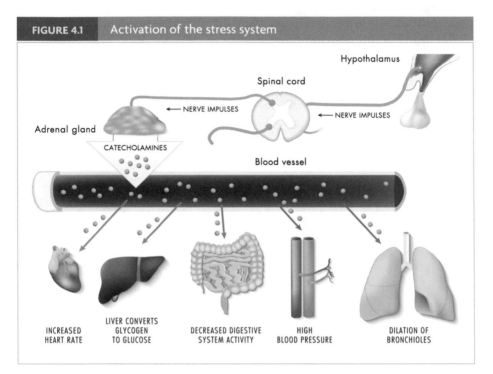

FIGURE 4.1   Activation of the stress system

Hypothalamus

Spinal cord

← NERVE IMPULSES   ← NERVE IMPULSES

Adrenal gland

CATECHOLAMINES

Blood vessel

| INCREASED HEART RATE | LIVER CONVERTS GLYCOGEN TO GLUCOSE | DECREASED DIGESTIVE SYSTEM ACTIVITY | HIGH BLOOD PRESSURE | DILATION OF BRONCHIOLES |

cold arise. The thyroid gland is usually affected at this stage. Infections become recurrent. More stimulants may be used to enhance energy and elevate mood.

STAGE 3: ADRENAL EXHAUSTION

If the stress isn't reduced, adrenal function will be further weakened because the body's need for cortisol remains unabated and the adrenals can't keep up with the demand. When a person reaches this stage, anxiety and exhaustion begin to appear simultaneously. Cortisol output gradually declines, and the body tries to conserve energy to ensure survival. This catabolic phase results in the breakdown of muscle tissue to produce energy. Chronic fatigue is common, exercise tolerance is reduced, and chronic fibromyalgia may appear. Toxic metabolites begin to accumulate throughout the body, leading to brain fog and insomnia. Depression intensifies and may become chronic. With a loss of homeostasis, the body enters into a state of disequilibrium. Without sufficient levels of hormones, the body begins to shut down nonessential functions to conserve energy in order to survive. Digestion slows and metabolic rate declines to conserve body weight. The afflicted individual may be unable to get out of bed or will have energy that lasts only briefly. The eventual result is a collapse of the HPA axis in which essential neuroendocrine feedback loops are unable to return the body's systems to homeostasis. Blood sugar levels plummet, and this leads to a further intolerance to stress as well as to increasing mental, physical, and emotional exhaustion. This stage is sometimes referred to as an "adrenal crash" or "adrenal burnout." When the symptoms of this stage interfere with day-to-day activities, the individual typically seeks medical treatment.

A hallucination is a fact, not an error; what is erroneous is a judgment based upon it.

BERTRAND RUSSELL (1872–1970)
British philosopher, logician, and social critic

STAGE 4: ADRENAL FAILURE

Although it rarely occurs, this final stage constitutes a total failure of the adrenal glands in response to stress. When people at this stage are confronted with a stressful situation, they are now susceptible to cardiovascular collapse and even death. The adrenals have largely ceased to function, and at this juncture there is little that can be done to restore the body's homeostasis. When adrenal fatigue has advanced to this point, the line between HPA axis dysfunction and adrenal insufficiency (Addison's disease) is muddled. Although the etiology of the two conditions differ, how they manifest clinically can be very similar (according to advocates of "adrenal fatigue"), as they both represent a corresponding low on the continuum of adrenal dysfunction. Symptoms may include sudden penetrating pain in the abdomen, legs, or lower back; severe diarrhea and vomiting; dehydration; low blood pressure; and loss of consciousness. If left untreated, the natural progression of this stage may be fatal.

Oh, how powerfully
the magnet of illusion attracts.

KARL FERDINAND GUTZKOW (1811–1878)

German novelist and journalist

Diagnosing "Adrenal Fatigue"

"A drenal fatigue" could be described as a cluster of symptoms that disrupts a person's regular ability to function. As yet, it can't be accounted for by a single pathognomonic marker or a medically acknowledged condition because the symptoms don't have a clear indication of etiology. Consequently, there isn't any one test that can confirm a diagnosis. Instead, so-called adrenal fatigue, like many other syndromes, is typically identified through a process of exclusion. This means that serious and medically recognized conditions must be ruled out as a cause for these diverse symptoms. Because the HPA axis can be affected by several chronic and/or metabolic disorders, other primary conditions must be excluded before intrinsic disorders of the HPA axis can be deemed responsible. When patients complain of symptoms, practitioners of conventional and complementary medicine typically order a range of tests, some of which may be conducted multiple times, and record every symptom reported. This requires not only experience but also a thorough knowledge of the various body systems. In addition, several office visits may be necessary before an accurate diagnosis can be made, so the process typically requires a fair amount of patience.

Screening for adrenal dysfunction may include standard hormone tests that measure cortisol and various thyroid hormone levels. To correctly make a diagnosis, a combination of lab testing, physical examinations with patient feedback, and questionnaires have been shown to be useful.

Be aware that a single measurement of cortisol levels or even a twenty-four-hour average is insufficient. The most accurate tests will take four individual samples at various points throughout the day and then map the cortisol levels over the course of a twenty-four-hour cycle. Because cortisol levels fluctuate dramatically from morning to night, it's important that health practitioners evaluate not only the average cortisol level but also the extent of the morning spike and how sharply it drops afterward.

For practitioners who aren't experienced with subclinical adrenal dysregulation or who don't acknowledge the existence of adrenal fatigue, interpreting the lab results can be tricky. That's because the reference ranges supplied by labs are so broad that typically only extremely low or extremely high cortisol levels are flagged. This underscores why using an optimal range rather than the reference range is so important. (See more about reference ranges on page 70.)

The primary lab test used to diagnose adrenal deficiency is one that measures cortisol levels. This may be done using blood, saliva, or urine, depending on the practitioner's preference and the patient's initial test results.

Most cortisol in the blood is bound to a protein; only a small percentage of it is "free" and biologically active. Blood cortisol testing evaluates both protein-bound and free cortisol while urine and salivary tests evaluate only free cortisol, which should correlate with the levels of free cortisol in the blood. Multiple blood and/or salivary cortisol levels collected at different times (such as morning, afternoon, and late at night) can be used to evaluate both cortisol levels and diurnal (daily) variation. A twenty-four-hour urine cortisol sample will not show diurnal variation; it will measure the total amount of unbound cortisol excreted in twenty-four hours.

The blood/serum test requires a blood sample, which is drawn through a needle from a vein in the arm. It's common to test serum cortisol twice in the same day—early in the morning and again around four o'clock in the afternoon.

A number of pharmaceuticals, especially oral contraceptives and any medicine that contains glucocorticoids or steroid hormones similar to cortisol, can affect cortisol levels, even after the medication has been discontinued. It's important for health-care practitioners to be fully informed about all the prescription and nonprescription medicines a patient is taking, including any herbs or supplements, prior to ordering or administering a test.

Cortisol levels may be higher than normal because of stress or physical trauma. Women in the last three months of pregnancy and highly trained athletes may have elevated cortisol levels. Other reasons cortisol levels may be higher than normal include alcoholism, depression, malnutrition, and panic disorder.

Patients may be asked to avoid strenuous physical activity the day before the test and may also be asked to lie down and relax for thirty minutes before the blood is drawn. Normal cortisol levels are usually highest early in the morning and lowest about midnight. However, this pattern will vary or be reversed if a person works rotating shifts or sleeps at different times on different days. If this diurnal change in cortisol levels doesn't occur, it may indicate overactive adrenal glands (Cushing's syndrome).

Because of how cortisol levels vary throughout the day, the timing of the test is very important. If a health-care provider suspects that too much cortisol is being produced, the test will probably be done late in the day. If the provider thinks that not enough cortisol is being made, the test will usually be done in the morning.

Numerous factors can affect the lab results, including the method each laboratory uses to do the test. Normal value ranges may vary slightly among different laboratories, depending on the type of test performed, specimens taken, and measurements used. (See "Interpreting Lab Results," page 72, for more information about this.)

Testing for Excess or Insufficient Cortisol Production

If lab results show a high blood cortisol level, the physician may order or conduct additional tests to confirm the level is actually abnormal and not merely a consequence of increased stress or the use of cortisol-like medication. These tests may include measuring the twenty-four-hour urinary cortisol, doing an overnight dexamethasone suppression test, and/or collecting a saliva sample before the patient goes to bed at night in order to measure cortisol at the time it should be the lowest. Urinary cortisol requires the collection of urine over a timed period, usually twenty-four hours. Since adrenocorticotropic hormone (ACTH) is secreted by the pituitary gland in pulses, this test helps determine whether the elevated blood cortisol level represents a true increase.

The dexamethasone suppression test involves analyzing a baseline sample for cortisol, then giving the patient oral dexamethasone (a synthetic glucocorticoid) and measuring cortisol levels in subsequent timed samples. Dexamethasone suppresses ACTH production and should decrease cortisol production if the source of the excess is stress.

Collecting a saliva sample to measure cortisol is a convenient way to determine whether the normal rhythm of cortisol production is failing. If one or more of these tests confirms abnormal cortisol production, then additional testing, including measuring ACTH, repeating the dexamethasone suppression test at higher doses, and radiologic imaging may be ordered.

If a physician suspects that the adrenal glands may not be producing adequate cortisol, or if the initial blood tests indicate insufficient cortisol production, an ACTH stimulation test may be ordered. This test involves measuring the level of cortisol in the patient's blood before and after the injection of synthetic ACTH. If the adrenal glands are functioning normally, cortisol levels will rise with the ACTH stimulation. If they are damaged or not functioning properly, the cortisol level will be low. A longer version of this test may be performed over one to three days to help distinguish between adrenal and pituitary insufficiency.

Reference Ranges

A reference range, also called a reference interval, is a set of values that includes upper and lower limits of a lab test based on a group of perceived healthy people. Through many years of research involving large, diverse populations, these ranges have become standardized, but the values in between those ranges may depend on a variety of factors, including age, sex, other characteristics, and type of specimen (such as blood, saliva, or urine). They can also be influenced by circumstantial conditions or behaviors, such as fasting or exercising prior to the test.

Health-care providers compare reference ranges to test results to determine a patient's current health status. But a test result on its own doesn't necessarily indicate illness, wellness, or risk for a health condition. It only becomes meaningful when taken into consideration along with other information about a patient, such as the results of a physical examination, current health status, reported symptoms, recent health changes, family and personal medical history, medication history, and other types of tests.

Most patients can now access their lab results online, but very few results can be properly understood by people who aren't health professionals. However, an experienced health-care provider can use reference ranges as a gauge to interpret the results and to help guide them in making the best decisions about managing a patient's health or treatment plan. A reference range is merely a starting point for health-care providers; they still need to make sense of the results in the context of a patient's medical history and current health presentation.

Laboratories report the patient's test results along with their (the lab's) reference ranges. Results that are out of range are typically highlighted or flagged and may include a comment when out-of-range results have clinical significance. Some reports include "critical values" that represent potentially life-threatening abnormalities. Every laboratory identifies certain key tests that have been associated with these life-threatening events, and critical values are required to be immediately reported to the health-care provider.

Depending on the information the health provider has already gathered about the patient's health status, a test result outside the normal range could help confirm a diagnosis, indicate the severity of a health problem, suggest a need for additional testing, or point to a need to reorder the test.

Interpreting Lab Results

L aboratory test results only have meaning when they're compared to reference ranges, which are the values expected for a healthy person. By comparing a patient's test results with reference values, a health-care provider can see if any of the test results fall outside the range of expected values. Values that are outside expected ranges can provide clues to help identify possible conditions or diseases.

Although the accuracy of laboratory tests has greatly improved over the past several decades, there can still be variability from lab to lab due to differences in testing equipment, chemical reagents, and techniques. Each laboratory establishes, or "validates," its own reference ranges by using data from its own equipment and methods, citing reference ranges from test manufacturers or other laboratories, or by testing a pool of perceived normal and healthy individuals. Consequently, a normal result in one lab may be considered abnormal in another. That's why, for the majority of lab tests, there is no single, universally applicable reference value.

The differences between reference ranges from different labs are usually not significant, but it's possible that one lab will report a result as being within range while another could report the same result as being out of range. That's why if a health condition is being monitored with lab tests, it's generally recommended to have the same lab perform the tests for consistency. Note that all clinical laboratories in the United States are periodically inspected as directed by federal guidelines and are subjected to an extensive review of quality control procedures.

The specific reference ranges that appear on a laboratory report are determined and provided by the laboratory that performed the test. While test results within normal limits may be a good sign, they aren't a guarantee of robust health. For many tests, there is a fair amount of overlap among results from healthy people and those who are sick, so there is still a chance there could be an undetected problem. The laboratory test results of some ill people often fall within the normal reference ranges, particularly during the early stages of a disease. At the same time, an abnormal test result doesn't necessarily indicate illness. Because many reference values are based on statistical ranges in healthy people, a healthy person could still be outside the statistical range. This is particularly true if the values are close to the expected normal range. However, an abnormal value can alert a health-care provider to a possible problem, especially if the test result is significantly outside the expected values.

Results that are far above or far below the reference range are a clear indication that further investigation is needed. But what about results that are only slightly above or slightly below the range? While healthy people sometimes have test results outside the range, for some conditions, test results that are even slightly out of range can be significant. A health-care provider may recommend follow-up testing to find out if the result of the repeated test shows normal ranges or persists in being outside the range.

Factors That Can Affect Test Results

Sundry factors can influence the outcome of laboratory test values. For example, technical errors can occur due to faulty processing or transporting of the specimen (exposure to heat, improper separation of red blood cells from plasma/serum, refrigeration problems). Circumstantial factors, such as something the person ate prior to the test or the person not fasting as instructed, recent physical exertion, not discontinuing medications or supplements, or not avoiding cigarettes or alcohol, may skew the results. A patient's compliance with test preparation instructions helps make a sample as close as possible to others, keeping it within the parameters of the reference group.

There are a few additional reasons why a test result could fall outside the established reference range, even if a patient is in good health. Usually these factors only have relevance when the test value is slightly higher or slightly lower than the reference range:

Biological variability. If a health-care provider runs the same test on a patient on several different occasions, there's a good chance that at least one of those times the result will fall outside the reference range, even though the patient may be healthy. That's because the body is constantly changing. Age, alcohol intake, diet, hormonal cycles, physical activity level, and even a change of season can cause alterations in the body's chemistry that can affect a test's result.

Individual variability. Reference ranges are usually established by collecting results from a large population and determining from the data a mean result (i.e., expected average) and a standard deviation (the expected variances from that average). There simply are some individuals who are healthy but whose typical test results don't fall within the expected range of the overall population.

Laboratory variability. If a health-care provider refers the patient to a different lab than was previously used for the patient's tests, an out-of-range result could be due to the new laboratory's testing methods, techniques, or reference ranges rather than caused by a significant change in the patient's health status.

Statistical variability. Reference ranges typically cover 95 percent of results for a healthy population. Statistically speaking, that means 5 percent of the people in that population will have results that fall outside the range limits.

Additional Tests

Several additional tests may be recommended by alternative health practitioners for patients reporting symptoms associated with presumed adrenal fatigue syndrome. However, most of these tests are based on little more than wishful thinking and speculation, not science. While physically harmless, be aware that they could mislead patients, offer false hope or unnecessary fear, and potentially delay treatment for more serious, underlying conditions.

Hair, tissue, mineral analysis (HTMA). Hair analysis is a test in which a sample of a person's hair (typically from the back of the neck) is sent to a laboratory for measurement of its mineral content. This test is often used by chiropractors, "nutritional consultants," and alternative health-care practitioners as a basis for prescribing supplements.

Iris contraction test (pupillary reflex). Normally the pupil of the eye will hold a steady contraction when it's exposed to light, which means that it will get smaller and will usually stay that way. This self-test measures the contraction of the iris in response to repeated exposure to dark light. Theoretically, in people with weakened adrenal function, the iris will be unable to maintain its contraction for very long. Alternatively, the pupil may not contract at all, or it might contract and then quickly dilate, or it might move from contraction to dilation.

To conduct the test, sit in front of a mirror in a darkened room. Take a weak flashlight or penlight and shine it across one eye from the side of your head, keeping the flashlight about six inches from your face (don't shine the light directly in the eye). According to the purported theory, if a person is in a hypoadrenal state (that is, their adrenal glands are underactive), the pupil will not be able to hold the contraction for longer than two minutes and will begin to dilate despite the light shining on it. In people with healthy adrenals, according to the theory, the contraction should last much longer.

Lower-than-normal body temperature. The normal human body temperature is 98 degrees F, but for some people the normal baseline temperature is lower. In addition, some people may notice a minor decrease in their normal body temperature as they age. What's "normal" may vary somewhat, depending on how, where, and when the temperature is taken. The are a number of possible causes for a lower-than-normal body temperature other than adrenal abnormalities, including acute infection, kidney disease, and hypothyroidism (which can slow the body's metabolism). If a person's body temperature has dropped to an unusually low level, medical help should be sought immediately.

Postural low blood pressure (Ragland's sign). When people who are in good health stand up, there is an almost immediate rise in blood pressure. Hypothetically, people who suffer from adrenal fatigue will see no change in their blood pressure upon standing or may even see a slight drop. Broadly speaking, the theory goes that the larger the drop in blood pressure, the more severe the case of adrenal fatigue.

Rogoff's sign. More of a symptom than a test, this refers to pain in the midback, where the ribs are located, that feels similar to a kidney infection, pulled muscle, or strained ligament.

Salivary hormone testing. Most salivary hormone tests are available online and can be obtained without a prescription. These tests measure the amount of free cortisol and dehydroepiandrosterone (DHEA), among other hormones, found in the saliva. Salivary hormone levels may vary according to the time of day the saliva is collected, the person's diet, or the person's level of hydration. Thus the timing of the saliva collection may affect the results, and the salivary flow rate can affect the concentration of certain hormones. Different laboratories may require different testing methods, such as obtaining several samples over a couple of weeks at specific times of the day. The results of these tests are often used to determine a supposed need for prescriptions of DHEA, vitamins, minerals, herbs, and other supplements.

The medical literature on salivary testing correlates salivary levels with serum levels, the gold standard of measurement. However, the medical literature fails to demonstrate that salivary tests alone are appropriate for screening, diagnosing, or monitoring patients with adrenal dysfunction. According to available guidelines, primary hypoadrenalism (Addison's disease) is suggested by markedly elevated plasma adrenocorticotropic hormone (ACTH) levels with low or normal serum cortisol levels. A diagnosis of adrenocortical insufficiency is established primarily by the use of the rapid ACTH stimulation test, which involves the assessment of the response of serum aldosterone and cortisol to ACTH infusion. Furthermore, there is inadequate evidence of the value of measuring salivary components to guide the prescription of supplement regimens. The clinical value of these tests depends not only on how well the salivary test corresponds to a serum test but also on the evidence of the effectiveness of the particular intervention that would be prescribed based on the results of the salivary test. Meta-analysis of the scientific literature shows that researchers question the value and validity of patients supplementing with DHEA to improve health outcomes.

White line test. This test is self-administered. Uncover the abdomen or the inner forearm for fifteen minutes so the skin can be seen in good light. Use the dull end of a ballpoint pen or a chopstick and lightly stroke the skin of the abdomen, making a mark about six inches in length; be sure not to scratch or break the skin's surface. Within a few seconds a line will appear. Theoretically, people with normal adrenal function will show an initial white line that will turn red in fifteen to twenty seconds, but if adrenal fatigue is present, the line will stay white for about two minutes and widen, but no red line will appear.

Adrenal Fatigue Questionnaire

The following informal questionnaire lists many symptoms commonly associated with adrenal fatigue syndrome. Although it's not intended to be an independent diagnostic tool and can't take the place of a comprehensive examination by a qualified clinician, these or similar questions are often used by alternative practitioners to determine the presence of supposed adrenal fatigue. If you like, use this questionnaire as a starting point to help you determine whether you might be at risk for adrenal impairment or another underlying condition, and whether you might benefit from further investigation by your doctor or health-care professional.

KEY SIGNS AND SYMPTOMS

YES	NO	I am chronically fatigued.
YES	NO	I wake up tired or unrefreshed, even after a good night's sleep.
YES	NO	My ability to handle stress and pressure has diminished.
YES	NO	I commonly experience mild to severe anxiety.
YES	NO	I commonly experience mild to severe depression.

YES	NO	I feel unwell most of the time.
YES	NO	I am less productive at work than I used to be.
YES	NO	My thinking seems foggy or confused, especially when I'm under pressure.
YES	NO	My moods fluctuate greatly.
YES	NO	I am often emotional and get upset easily.
YES	NO	I become anxious when I'm under pressure.
YES	NO	I suffer from muscle weakness and aches and pains.
YES	NO	My ankles are swollen, especially in the evening.
YES	NO	I have restless legs syndrome.
YES	NO	I sometimes feel weak all over.
YES	NO	I often get nervous indigestion.
YES	NO	My skin and/or hair are dry and thinning.
YES	NO	My nails are thin and brittle.
YES	NO	I have dark circles under my eyes.
YES	NO	My libido (sex drive) is greatly diminished.
YES	NO	I get dizzy when I stand up quickly.
YES	NO	I have frequent unexplained headaches.
YES	NO	I am frequently cold or have a decreased tolerance for cold.
YES	NO	I have low blood pressure.
YES	NO	I often have feelings of hopelessness and despair.
YES	NO	I often feel on edge, pessimistic, impatient, or irritable.
YES	NO	I need to lie down after periods of emotional pressure or stress.

PREDISPOSING CONDITIONS

YES	NO	I've taken large or long-term doses of corticosteroids or anti-inflammatory drugs.
YES	NO	I have an autoimmune disease or another inflammatory condition.
YES	NO	I have post-traumatic stress syndrome (PTSD).
YES	NO	I have a history of childhood sexual, emotional, or physical abuse.

YES	NO	I have experienced severe stress or long periods of stress in the past.
YES	NO	I have a history of alcoholism and/or drug abuse.
YES	NO	I have one or more chronic illnesses or diseases.

LIFESTYLE PATTERNS

YES	NO	I am overwhelmed by my responsibilities.
YES	NO	My work or personal life is constantly stressful.
YES	NO	I occasionally drive myself to the point of exhaustion.
YES	NO	My relationships at home or at work are unsatisfactory.
YES	NO	I have poor dietary habits.
YES	NO	I don't exercise regularly.
YES	NO	I don't have enjoyable hobbies or activities.
YES	NO	I have little control over how I spend my time.

SLEEP AND ENERGY PATTERNS

YES	NO	I am easily fatigued. I often suddenly run out of energy.
YES	NO	I struggle to keep up with life's daily demands.
YES	NO	I have difficulty getting up in the morning and prefer to sleep in late.
YES	NO	My most refreshing sleep is between 7:00 and 9:00 a.m.
YES	NO	I have low energy before a meal but feel better after I eat.
YES	NO	I often experience an afternoon drop in energy.
YES	NO	I often have to force myself to keep going during a long or busy day.
YES	NO	I feel my best after 6:00 p.m.
YES	NO	I usually do my best work late at night or in the wee hours of the morning.
YES	NO	I am typically tired between 9:00 and 10:00 p.m., but I resist going to bed.
YES	NO	It often takes me longer than fifteen minutes to fall asleep at night.
YES	NO	I usually get a second burst of energy around 11:00 p.m. that can last from 1:00 to 2:00 a.m.

YES	NO	I often feel tired after exercising rather than energized.
YES	NO	I have trouble staying asleep. I often wake up in the middle of the night.

HEALTH EVENTS

YES	NO	I have multiple chemical sensitivities.
YES	NO	I have chronic fatigue syndrome.
YES	NO	I have rheumatoid arthritis.
YES	NO	I have fibromyalgia.
YES	NO	I have asthma.
YES	NO	I have Raynaud's syndrome.
YES	NO	I have numerous food sensitivities or allergies.
YES	NO	I have many environmental sensitivities or allergies.
YES	NO	I have insomnia or difficulty sleeping or staying asleep.
YES	NO	I am prone to colds and flu.
YES	NO	I frequently get rashes, dermatitis, or other skin conditions.
YES	NO	I have gum infections and/or tooth problems or abscesses.

DIETARY PATTERNS

YES	NO	I need caffeinated coffee or other stimulants to get going in the morning.
YES	NO	I need coffee, colas, chocolate, sugar, or high-fat foods to stay energized throughout the day.
YES	NO	I drink more than eight ounces of coffee, tea, soda, or other caffeinated beverages every day.

YES	NO	I eat at irregular times.
YES	NO	I often crave and indulge in salty foods.
YES	NO	I need to snack frequently to avoid feeling weak or light-headed.
YES	NO	I become shaky, irritable, or sick if I skip a meal.
YES	NO	I crave sweet foods, desserts, and pastries.

SOURCES OF RELIEF

YES	NO	Regular meals help reduce the severity of my symptoms.
YES	NO	I feel better almost immediately after a stressful situation is resolved.
YES	NO	Spending time with friends, especially at night, makes me feel better.
YES	NO	I often feel better when I take naps or lie down for a while.
YES	NO	My symptoms improve when stress levels are lower, such as during a vacation or time away from work.

The purpose of this questionnaire is for you to see how many of these symptoms you have. There are a total of eighty-one questions. The more questions you responded to with a "yes" answer, the more likely it is an alternative health practitioner would diagnose you with adrenal fatigue. Note that many people who are healthy may still experience a number of these symptoms. If you have twenty or fewer of these indicators and your symptoms don't include chronic fatigue or a decreased ability to handle stress, it's less likely that an alternative health practitioner would diagnose you with adrenal fatigue syndrome. If you have severe depression, anxiety, or feelings of hopelessness or despair, please contact a health professional immediately, as these could indicate a serious condition that requires urgent attention.

Illness is the night side of life,
a more onerous citizenship.
Everyone who is born holds dual citizenship,
in the kingdom of the well
and in the kingdom of the sick.
Although we all prefer to use the good passport,
sooner or later each of us is obliged,
at least for a spell, to identify ourselves
as citizens of that other place.

SUSAN SONTAG
Illness as Metaphor

The "Adrenal Fatigue" Conundrum

META-ANALYSIS OF CURRENT RESEARCH

A recent systematic review of the scientific literature concluded that there was no evidence to support the theory of adrenal fatigue as an actual medical condition. Even so, alternative health-care practitioners, a handful of medical doctors, and the general public persist in using the term "adrenal fatigue" to describe the cluster of symptoms believed to be caused by chronic exposure to stress and stressful situations. However, the condition has not been recognized by the Endocrine Society, a global organization representing over eighteen thousand endocrinologists from 122 countries. The Endocrine Society asserts that adrenal fatigue is not a true medical condition and contends that there are no scientific facts to support the theory that long-term mental, emotional, or physical stress drains the adrenal glands or causes the variety of symptoms that have come to be associated with that term.

Nevertheless, a few medical societies, although none that are recognized by the American Board of Medical Specialties or the Association of American Medical Colleges, claim that adrenal fatigue is both a real and underdiagnosed condition. According to these societies, screening for adrenal fatigue in patients typically includes a comprehensive questionnaire (similar to the one on pages 77–81) and tests for basal (morning) serum cortisol levels and circadian salivary cortisol levels. Patients who present impaired levels from these tests are then typically treated with supplements and corticosteroids (primarily hydrocortisone), regardless of the etiology of the impairment. As a result, supplements and corticosteroids are likely being prescribed unnecessarily to a large number of patients, which could be dangerous.

Arguments in favor of using corticosteroids as a treatment for alleged adrenal fatigue include the immediate and significant improvement of symptoms in patients taking the hormones. In addition, some providers allege that the criteria used by endocrinologists to prescribe corticosteroids are too strict, and that if alternative practitioners didn't offer the hormones to their patients, many sufferers wouldn't receive adequate treatment. Nonetheless, there are equally compelling and logical arguments against routine corticosteroid use for these patients. First, corticosteroids promote a sense of well-being, although usually temporary, regardless of the condition being treated, so almost all patients who take them are going to report feeling better, especially initially. Second, even at low doses, corticosteroids increase the risk of several disorders: cardiovascular diseases, glaucoma, metabolic disorders, myopathy (a disease of muscle tissues), osteoporosis, psychiatric disorders, and sleep disturbances. Third, if people take adrenal hormone supplements when they don't need them, the adrenal glands may stop working and become unable to make these essential hormones when their bodies are under physical stress and desperately need them. And finally, when these supplements are discontinued, the person's adrenal glands can remain dormant for months, which could result in the development of adrenal crisis (see page 30), a life-threatening condition.

Science versus Subjectivity

Is adrenal fatigue syndrome real? The answer isn't simple, and it probably depends on who you ask. But as yet, there is no substantiation in the scientific literature to prove its existence. The reported symptoms of adrenal fatigue are, for the most part, broad and unspecific. While the symptoms themselves are no doubt real, they easily overlap with other known medical issues. But the primary concern is that the reported symptoms are not objective or measurable by current methodologies. In other words, there are no valid tests or reliable symptom scores to assess how mild or severe a case may be. Consequently, without any means to accurately measure the severity of the "syndrome," there are no ways to accurately measure the effectiveness of any treatments that may be prescribed for it.

There are a number of questions all practitioners should be seeking answers to in order to determine whether adrenal fatigue is an actual disorder:

- Is fatigue actually related to demonstrably depleted adrenal function?
- Do fatigued but otherwise healthy patients present relative adrenal failure?
- Are the adrenal glands associated with the pathophysiology of fatigue in diseases?
- Which tests were performed to establish markers or triggers of adrenal dysregulation or failure?

Theories on adrenal impairment as the source of fatigue are alluring because they offer up a treatable condition; it's simply human nature to want to make sense of patterns and clusters of symptoms and attempt to label them. But it's critical to determine whether there's a true correlation between adrenal status and fatigue states or fatigue-related diseases and to examine the results of any peer-reviewed studies correlating cortisol and fatigue. It turns out that only a handful of citations in the scientific literature have been found using the expression "adrenal fatigue," and these were merely descriptive; they weren't reporting on any tests performed regarding the HPA axis and supposed adrenal fatigue. Instead, studies that have tried to connect HPA axis dysregulation with fatigue have used the term "burnout" to denote verifiable adrenal depletion.

Obviously there is a divide between the terminology used in the scientific literature and that used by alternative practitioners and the general public regarding this supposed condition. Because the term "adrenal fatigue" has already been stigmatized and is lacking the proper scientific support, it makes sense that a more suitable, accurate, and widely accepted name should be given to the purported condition. In addition, the methodology used to evaluate any connection between adrenal fatigue and adrenal function should be standardized among clinicians and medical associations that contend that adrenal impairment occurs in patients with fatigue before evidence of clinical hypocortisolism manifests, as this would strengthen any proof of a causal correlation should one eventually be found.

There currently are no approved, reliable, or consistent methods to clinically screen for alleged adrenal fatigue. Although validated surveys have been used in studies that investigated fatigue states, they weren't correlated with proper cortisol assessment methods. The Trier Social Stress Test (TSST), developed at the University of Trier in Germany, is currently the only credible survey that's been formally tested and standardized as a trigger of stress. It has become a standard protocol for the experimental induction of moderate psychological stress in psychobiological research and could contribute to the valuable understanding of the role of various biological pathways involved in stress-related disorders and the developmental variability of the stress response. The TSST has been found to reliably activate the HPA stress axis and to trigger a two- to threefold release of the stress hormone cortisol (compared to non-stress control conditions) in 70–80 percent of participants, which sheds light on some of the multiple variables that contribute to adrenocortical stress responses. Moreover, various other indicators confirm the stress-inducing potential of the TSST, including changes in cardiovascular parameters and high levels of self-reported stress and anxiety.

Functional tests (those that identify, interpret, and quantify systems of dysfunction) are the only methods endorsed by endocrinology societies to assess adrenal cortisol production. But there has been conflicting data using these tests when trying to differentiate exhausted, fatigued individuals from healthy patients, such as an unexpected increase (rather than decrease) in cortisol levels in fatigued subjects in the selected studies, rendering these methods unusable in terms of differentiating fatigued from non-fatigued individuals.

An important consideration is whether cortisol markers can be used to assess cortisol impairment. Major tests used to identify underlying causes of the fatigue state have been unable to demonstrate significant differences or causality in heterogeneous groups of subjects, since the etiology and pathogenesis of fatigue status could be the consequence of other disorders, such as sleep disturbances.

Adrenal size could be considered another marker of adrenal activity, as the enlargement of the adrenal glands could be the result of ACTH overstimulation by the pituitary glands, and an atrophic (diminished) gland may reflect adrenal insufficiency at any level of the HPA axis. However, there has been little to no research to date in which adrenal size has been checked in fatigued or exhausted patients. Similarly, although levels of DHEA-S (the sulfated form of DHEA) could also be a potential marker for adrenal atrophy or dysfunction, it's still uncertain whether it plays any pathophysiological role in fatigue. Finally, none of these as yet has been shown to be an accurate marker of fatigue, and studies haven't correlated them with HPA axis dysfunction as an etiology of fatigue.

An extensive meta-analysis conducted by endocrinologists to examine a possible correlation between the HPA axis, "adrenal fatigue," and other conditions associated with fatigue, exhaustion, or burnout has been unable to demonstrate the existence of adrenal fatigue. In order for adrenal fatigue to be substantiated, further investigation is required by the groups that claim it exists, and those studies must employ the most appropriate scientific methods to assess the correlation between stress, fatigue, and the HPA axis.

Fact versus Fake

How can you tell when a theorized syndrome is an actual medical condition? A true medical condition is a distinct clinical entity with something specific about one or more of the symptoms or combination of symptoms. A collection of common, nonspecific symptoms doesn't constitute a clinical entity. A specific biomarker, such as a laboratory test or study that confirms an abnormal result that will respond to specific treatment, also provides validity.

"Fake" diseases are fabricated without any objective, empirical evidence to confirm their existence. They emerge from vague symptoms that can't be attributed to any particular medical condition, giving an alternative health provider broad leeway in providing a fictitious diagnosis and treatment plan, even if the condition is completely unsubstantiated or possibly made up. Because a diagnosis guides the treatment plan (or ought to), it's essential to get the diagnosis right. That means running proven tests to rule out serious illness rather than a practitioner jumping to a preferred diagnosis and treatment, which is frequently the case when it comes to adrenal fatigue.

Fraudulent syndromes are often confirmed by laboratory tests that are misused or misinterpreted to provide bogus legitimacy for a questionable diagnosis. For instance, these tests may be designed to produce false positives, while medically valid tests with verifiable diagnostic criteria may be dismissed as inappropriate or ill-advised. In the case of adrenal fatigue, highly variable tests, such as the saliva test for cortisol, might be given many times until the practitioner obtains the desired result. This type of test is ideal for generating false positives, so it's popular among advocates of adrenal fatigue.

At this time the only "evidence" proffered by adrenal fatigue specialists is anecdotal. Typically when the patient makes a few healthy lifestyle changes in conjunction with either real or dubious treatment, and positive outcomes result, the dubious treatment receives the credit. The story might unfold along these lines: "I was tired and depressed, but my regular physician found nothing wrong with me. Then I went to Dr. X and was diagnosed with adrenal fatigue. Following Dr. X's advice, I changed my diet, began exercising, and worked on controlling my stress. I also took Dr. X's magic tonic every day. I was shocked how well the magic tonic worked! One year later, I'm feeling great!"

Real diseases and syndromes, along with the treatments for them, are supported by a body of scientific literature. But dubious practitioners with self-invented (and often self-serving) diagnoses and conspiracy theories about how dreadful conventional medicine is and how fabulous their alternative treatments are don't have a scientific foundation. That's not to say that mainstream medicine doesn't have its faults and failings. Inarguably, it's not perfect. However, that's not a good reason to accept unsubstantiated, misleading, and potentially harmful claims.

Neurotics complain of their illness, but they make the most of it, and when it comes to taking it away from them, they will defend it like a lioness her young.

SIGMUND FREUD (1856–1939)
Austrian neurologist and the founder of psychoanalysis

But what about other legitimate medical diagnoses that aren't yet detectable by tests? Diagnoses such as dementia, depression, irritable bowel syndrome, and Parkinson's disease are often determined and treated based on symptoms, not the results of lab tests. While that's certainly true, many fabricated syndromes are used to exploit susceptible people who are merely dealing with common symptoms that are the fallout of contemporary life. Some of these individuals may actually have a real underlying disease, but they may get distracted from investigating an authentic diagnosis when a fake one is readily offered up instead. For many people, lifestyle adjustments are all they need to improve their health, and that may be the best place for them to focus their efforts, rather than on magic supplements and elixirs to treat syndromes that are not yet confirmed and may very well be fictitious.

Myth versus Truth

MYTH: *Adrenal fatigue is caused by extreme, chronic, or prolonged stress.*

TRUTH: There currently is no scientific evidence that supports the theory that long-term mental, emotional, or physical stress drains the adrenal glands or causes HPA axis dysregulation.

MYTH: *Adrenal fatigue is a medical condition.*

TRUTH: No scientific proof currently exists to support the theory that adrenal fatigue is a true medical condition. Doctors are concerned that if patients are told they have this condition, the underlying cause of their symptoms may not be found or a proper diagnosis may be delayed. Also, any treatment for supposed adrenal fatigue may be expensive, since insurance companies are unlikely to cover the costs.

MYTH: *Adrenal fatigue can be measured and diagnosed using a salivary cortisol test.*

TRUTH: The salivary cortisol test is a way to measure the body's adaptation to stress and is useful for helping to diagnose adrenal insufficiency (see page 23), as long as it's used in conjunction with other recommended tests. However, salivary cortisol is not necessarily representative of blood cortisol, and numerous factors may influence the saliva reading, making it an unreliable biomarker of stress on its own.

MYTH: *Various tests can confirm a diagnosis of adrenal fatigue.*

TRUTH: Adrenal insufficiency is a recognized medical disease that occurs when the adrenal glands cannot produce enough hormones. It's caused by damage to the adrenal glands or a problem with the pituitary gland. Adrenal insufficiency is a rare condition that is diagnosed through blood tests, but there is no single test or group of tests that can detect alleged adrenal fatigue. Often a person is told he or she has adrenal fatigue based on symptoms alone. Sometimes a blood or saliva test may be recommended, but tests for adrenal fatigue are not based on scientific fact or supported by scientific studies, so the results and interpretation of these tests may not be substantiated. Because there are no tests to confirm or disconfirm the condition, it's not possible for health practitioners to determine what might be classified as adrenal fatigue and what might not be.

MYTH: *Existing blood tests simply are not sensitive enough to detect small declines in adrenal function.*

TRUTH: While it's quite possible this may be true, there currently is no evidence to support such a theory.

MYTH: *Symptoms of adrenal fatigue are all in a person's head.*

TRUTH: Reported symptoms of adrenal fatigue are generally broad and nonspecific and overlap with known medical conditions. Because symptoms are subjective, they aren't measurable. However, that doesn't mean the symptoms aren't real.

For a while she considered being ill, but she changed her mind.

TOVE JANSSON, *The Summer Book*

MYTH: *There are proven protocols for treating adrenal fatigue.*

TRUTH: Because there is no way to accurately test for or measure supposed adrenal fatigue, practitioners have no evidence that it actually exists, or if it does, no way to assess how mild or severe a case may be. For this reason, they also have no way to verify when the condition has been corrected or resolved.

7

The question is
not how to get cured,
but how to live.

JOSEPH CONRAD (1857–1924)
Polish-British writer and novelist

Next Steps

or people who constantly feel unwell, it's incredibly frustrating to have a doctor be unable or unwilling to discover their true problem. That's completely understandable, because the symptoms a patient is experiencing are real. Indeed, that's why people often turn to alternative practitioners and why alternative practitioners often label their patients' cluster of symptoms as adrenal fatigue. A tangible diagnosis gives patients hope that whatever they're dealing with can be cured. It also opens the door for these same health-care providers to sell untested, unproven supplements to optimistic, impressionable, or desperate patients and profit from them. However, with no scientific evidence to substantiate the concept of adrenal fatigue, and with no reliable method of detecting, measuring, or resolving it, it's impossible to make such a diagnosis, or at least one that's valid, or recommend therapies or prescribe appropriate remedies. If a comparable scenario played out with other common medical conditions, such as high blood pressure or type 2 diabetes, the doctor would have no way of knowing when to increase, decrease, or stop the patient's medication. It's like aiming at a moving target when you're blindfolded—there's a near-zero chance you'll hit your mark. At what point do any potential benefits of unwarranted or spurious treatments outweigh the risks and expense?

Nevertheless, a diagnosis of adrenal fatigue could have some unexpected advantages. When people have a specific reason to take action and adjust their lifestyles, improve their diets, and reduce their stressors, they're often motivated to do so. That's one reason so many individuals with supposed adrenal fatigue who are given a treatment plan that includes positive lifestyle changes end up experiencing improvement and feeling better.

But what if the real issue is deeper and more complex than simply poor diet and high stress? Accepting adrenal fatigue as the primary reason for symptoms can be dangerous because it will prolong the time required to discover what's actually the root cause. Conventional doctors urge patients to not waste precious time accepting an unproven diagnosis of adrenal fatigue. Instead, they encourage anyone who is feeling exhausted, weak, chronically ill, hopeless, or sad to obtain a medically accepted diagnosis so the true source of those symptoms—such as adrenal insufficiency, depression, obstructive sleep apnea, or other health problems—can be properly explored and treated.

Practitioners who support the notion of adrenal fatigue may advise their patients to make important lifestyle adjustments, such as giving up alcohol, drugs, caffeine, and smoking. They may also suggest starting an exercise program, eating healthier foods, and following a regular daily routine for sleeping and waking. These types of lifestyle changes almost always help people feel better, no matter what medical diagnosis they've been given. But these practitioners may also encourage their patients to undergo various tests or buy special supplements and vitamins that the practitioners themselves have formulated or that they claim have been developed specifically for adrenal health and support. People who don't feel well are yearning for answers and solutions, which makes them easy prey for naïve, inexperienced, or shady practitioners who may be eager to sell these unproven, expensive, and even potentially harmful tests, supplements, and treatments. Although some ordinary vitamins and minerals might be health supportive for certain conditions, taking supplements sold as a treatment for adrenal fatigue could be risky. Nutrition supplements should be used to address known deficiencies linked with particular conditions, but only a handful of scientific studies even mention the term "adrenal fatigue," let alone have tested for associated nutrient deficiencies.

The US Food and Drug Administration (the governmental arm that oversees most food and medical products in the United States) doesn't regulate nutritional supplements and vitamins. This means there's no guarantee that what's on the label of a supplement is actually what's inside the bottle. Laboratory testing has shown that some supplements have very few, if any, active ingredients, and in others the dose of a particular ingredient has been found to be too high. This is often the case if the supplements are purchased from a compounding pharmacy, where they are made directly by the pharmacist. There are also many hormone supplements available that promise to treat adrenal fatigue, but taking adrenal hormone supplements when they aren't needed can do far more harm than good and may instigate adrenal crisis (see page 30), a potentially life-threatening condition.

Getting an accurate and legitimate diagnosis is crucial for any person who feels ill or whose well-being has been compromised. Even though it's disheartening for patients to have symptoms that defy diagnosis, heeding advice from unqualified practitioners can be ineffective at best and dangerous or even deadly at worst. Beware of any website or practitioner that diagnoses an illness and also sells the cure.

Whether or not adrenal fatigue exists, taking measures to improve your diet, overhaul harmful habits, and better manage life's stressors are the safest and surest keys to regaining your health. And there definitely are proven methods to do each of these that will benefit almost anyone who has received a diagnosis of "adrenal fatigue," or even people who have received a clean bill of health from their doctors despite experiencing many of the symptoms commonly associated with alleged adrenal fatigue. Although changing ingrained patterns and lifelong habits requires more effort, diligence, and discipline than popping a pill or taking a potion, the upshot is a stronger body and healthier mind so you can endure and overcome the challenges life throws at you.

Stress Management

Stress is at the core of presumed adrenal fatigue because it's the body's response to stress that ignites the flow of "stress hormones" from the HPA axis, and it's the resolution of stress that signals negative feedback loops to halt that hormonal release. Consequently, knowing how to manage stress levels is the crucial first step to getting a handle on any potential health issues associated with possible stress-related hormone imbalances, "adrenal fatigue," or HPA axis dysfunction.

Contemporary life is teeming with stress, and it may seem as though there's little we can do to minimize it. Bills pile up, we need more hours in the day, and work and home responsibilities are relentless. But you actually have more control over stress than you may realize. At the heart of stress management is learning how to effectively master bad habits, handle obsessive thoughts and emotions, and take charge of problems. Regardless of how stressful life seems, there are steps we all can take to relieve the pressure, regain control, restore our health, and reclaim our lives.

While there's currently no scientific evidence that stress depletes our adrenal hormones or causes damage to the adrenal glands or the HPA axis, there's no question that living with high levels of stress can take a toll on our health and put our emotional equilibrium and overall well-being in jeopardy. Chronic stress clouds our thinking, impedes our ability to function, and hinders our ability to enjoy life.

However, effective stress management can break the hold stress has on our lives so we can be happier, healthier, and more productive. The ultimate goal is balance: achieving the resilience to stand up to pressure and meet life's challenges head on while ensuring sufficient time and energy for work, relationships, relaxation, and fun. But stress management is not a one-size-fits-all approach. It's important to explore and experiment to discover what works best for you and your individual needs, preferences, and circumstances.

First, try to identify your stressors. While major life events (such as buying a house or going through a divorce) tend to be obvious, the sources of chronic stress are usually far more subtle and complicated. Pay attention to how you react to difficult situations and how your stress levels increase because of negative self-talk and harmful beliefs or attitudes. In many ways we're often responsible for contributing to ongoing stress and are our own worst enemies. But the upside of this is that we can be equally instrumental in changing our response to stressful situations. If we have a hand in worsening our stress levels, then it's also within our power to improve them.

Second, adopt healthy coping strategies. Take a look at how you respond to the stressors in your life so you can determine whether your approaches are healthy and helpful or obstructive and damaging. If your current methods of dealing with stress aren't supporting your emotional and physical health, it's crucial that you find other ways of coping that are more constructive. You can experiment with a wide range of approaches to discover which ones fit your needs and help you calm down and feel in control. The suggestions in this chapter will give you a good start in finding options to explore.

Change Your Response to Stressful Situations

Although you can't control your autonomic nervous system's response to stress, there are some stressors in life you can anticipate and prepare for. When those arise, you can either avoid or change the situation or alter your response to it by following these tips:

Reclaim your power. While it's never wise to evade responsibilities or dodge a situation that needs to be addressed, when circumstances are unworkable or you've reached the breaking point, it's essential to take back your power or walk away. Discover how much you can handle and what your limit is. Differentiate between what you think you *ought* to do and what you truly *need* to do. Learn how to say no and stand your ground.

Limit stressful experiences. If certain people or situations make you feel anxious, uncomfortable, or on edge, you don't have to be involved with them. Minimize the time you spend with toxic individuals, especially your time alone with them, or sever your relationship, if that's the only realistic solution. Avoid stress-producing experiences whenever possible. If you know something will upset you (such as reading about current events or watching a scary movie), find more calming, soothing options.

icate. Discussing what you're feeling or going through can narkable stress reliever, even if there isn't anything you can nange the situation. If you don't have someone you trust to talk with, make an appointment with a therapist or write down your thoughts in a journal. Bottling up emotions is not only unhealthy, but it also feeds feelings of anger and bitterness that could lead to hostility, violent behavior, or depression. If someone or something is annoying you, speak up rather than holding in your feelings and letting resentment build. Learn how to communicate your concerns in a manner that's honest, respectful, and constructive.

Laugh about it. A sense of humor in trying times releases tension, decreases levels of stress hormones, lowers blood pressure, reduces anxiety, and helps maintain perspective. Sometimes just laughing about the absurdity of a situation is all that's needed to get you through it. (See "Humor Therapy," page 17.)

Accept what you can't change. Many aspects of life are beyond our control, including what other people say and do. Often the best way to cope with adversity is to simply accept things as they are. While there's no doubt that acceptance may be difficult, in the long run it's easier than railing against an immutable situation. Rather than letting your circumstances stress you out, focus on what you *can* control, such as how you respond to the difficult people, problems, and challenges in your life.

Move Your Body

Although exercise may be one of the last things you feel like doing when you're stressed out, moderate physical activity is among the top best stress relievers. In addition to being a valuable distraction from daily worries, exercise releases endorphins, the "feel good" hormones that enhance mood and boost energy. Exercise also reduces anxiety and depression and enhances sleep.

You don't have to become an athlete or spend hours at the gym to reap the benefits of movement. While exercising for thirty minutes five to seven days a week will provide the greatest benefits, you can build up your fitness level gradually or distribute your activity in small increments throughout the day, such as in two fifteen-minute sessions or three ten-minute sessions. Even a single ten-minute walk would be beneficial. The first step, though, is to just get started.

Making exercise a habit takes more than just knowing how and why to do it; it requires the right mind-set and an intelligent approach. Whatever your age or fitness level, there are measures you can take to make exercise less intimidating and more fun and instinctive. A little exercise is better than none at all. In fact, adding just small amounts of physical activity to your daily routine can have an enormous positive effect on your emotional well-being. Start slowly and be gentle with yourself. Try not to be discouraged by what you can't do; focus on consistency instead. You'll be amazed at how quickly you'll see improvements in your mood and energy levels.

Exercise can be used as a form of "meditation in action," as with yoga and tai chi (see page 116). Zeroing in on how your body feels as you move and noticing the rhythm of your breath and the flexing of your muscles will not only improve your physical conditioning but will also divert your attention away from negative thoughts and worries, further helping to ease stress and anxiety.

If you're not the type of person who likes to follow a structured exercise program, try thinking about physical activity as a lifestyle choice rather than as a task that must be crossed off your to-do list. Examine your daily routine and look for ways to slip in a bit of extra movement. Even small activities will add up over the course of the day. Housework, gardening, and yard work can be considered exercise too, especially if they're done at a lively pace.

Additional Stress-Relief Approaches

Although stress management can't cure physical illness, it can play a vital role in medical treatments. Specific stress-reduction strategies tend to target specific medical conditions, but in general, the quality of life and well-being of almost anyone will improve when stress is reduced. Bear in mind that what works for one person may not necessarily work for someone else or for you. Also note that some stress-reduction approaches may not be medically approved or have scientific validity, even though many people claim they work for them. Be aware that no single method is always successful; usually a combination of approaches is what turns out to be the most effective.

A number of relaxation exercises can help you to become more aware of muscle tension and other physical sensations of stress. Once you know what the stress response feels like in your body, you can make a conscious effort to practice a relaxation exercise as soon as you start to feel stress symptoms arise. Catching and alleviating stress early on can help prevent it from spiraling out of control.

The more you practice specific stress-reduction techniques, the better you will become at them. Be patient and don't let your efforts to relax turn into yet another stressor. If one stress-relief exercise doesn't seem to work for you, try another. Here are just a few of the many strategies you can explore:

ACUPRESSURE

Acupressure is the practice of applying precise pressure, usually with the fingertips, to various tactical points on the body. The objective is to balance a person's energy, or life force, called "qi" in traditional Chinese medicine or "chi" in the West. The pressure points lie along channels of energy in the body known as meridians. Acupressure therapy can be used to relieve pain, reduce muscle tension, improve circulation, and promote deep states of relaxation. It may also be used to treat specific conditions, such as chronic fatigue, emotional stress, fibromyalgia, migraine headaches, motion sickness, nausea and vomiting, and neck and back pain. Although acupressure is usually provided by massage therapists and other types of bodyworkers, it can also be learned as a self-care technique that individuals can perform on themselves.

ACUPUNCTURE

Acupuncture is a holistic treatment mechanism based on traditional Chinese medicine and the traditions of Japan, Korea, and other countries. It involves the stimulation of strategic locations on the body by inserting thin, solid metallic needles into the skin. Sometimes heat, pressure, or mild electrical current is used along with the needles. Surprisingly, although needles are used in acupuncture, the treatments are relatively pain-free. Acupuncturists believe that illness occurs when something is blocking or imbalancing a person's life energy (known as "qi" or "chi"), and acupuncture is a way to unblock or influence it to flow back into balance. One of the most popular uses of acupuncture is for reducing chronic pain, depression, anxiety, and stress without the need for medications, which often cause unwanted side effects.

AROMATHERAPY

Aromatherapy is the therapeutic application of naturally extracted aromatic plant oils, known as essential oils, to promote physical and psychological health. Essential oils are concentrated volatile extracts taken from the roots, leaves, seeds, or blossoms of plants. Although aromatherapy oils are commonly inhaled using a diffuser, steam bath, or spray to disperse oil droplets into the air, they may also be diluted with a neutral base (such as a lotion or cream) or neutral carrier oil (such as sweet almond oil or olive oil) and applied topically or massaged into the skin. Note that essential oils should not be applied directly to the skin without first being diluted; a few drops of essential oil to an ounce of carrier oil is the usual concentration. Never take essentials oils by mouth, as some oils are toxic and ingesting them could be fatal.

BIOFEEDBACK

Biofeedback therapy is a noninvasive, drug-free technique that helps patients learn how to control body processes that are normally involuntary, such as blood pressure, heart rate, or muscle tension. Patients are connected to electrical sensors that provide feedback about the body's functions that can help them focus on making subtle changes to achieve the desired results, such as relaxing certain muscles to help reduce pain. Essentially biofeedback gives people the power to use their thoughts to control their bodies to improve various health conditions through teaching relaxation techniques and mental exercises that can alleviate symptoms. Therapists may use several different biofeedback methods depending on the patient's particular health problems and objectives. Although biofeedback therapy and training are available at physical therapy clinics, medical centers, and hospitals, a growing number of biofeedback devices and programs are also being marketed for home use.

COGNITIVE BEHAVIORAL THERAPY

Cognitive behavioral therapy was invented by psychiatrist Aaron Beck in the 1960s. It's a short-term, goal-oriented approach that basically combines psychotherapy with behavioral therapy. The objective is to modify ingrained behavior or patterns of thinking that contribute to people's problems and, by doing so, change the way they feel. Cognitive behavioral therapy is used to treat a wide range of ailments, such as anxiety, depression, drug and alcohol abuse, insomnia, and even relationship problems. It works by helping people focus on their cognitive processes—that is, their attitudes, thoughts, and beliefs—so they can learn how these processes affect their behavioral and emotional responses.

DEEP BREATHING

Also called slow abdominal breathing, belly breathing, diaphragmatic breathing, and paced respiration, deep breathing occurs when the air coming through the nose fully fills the lungs and causes the lower part of the belly to rise. Similar to conscious breathing (see page 13), deep breathing is the opposite of "chest breathing," which is the way most people tend to breathe. Chest breathing increases tension and anxiety, whereas deep breathing releases tension and reduces anxiety. That's because shallow chest breathing limits the diaphragm's range of motion, and the lowest part of the lungs doesn't get its full share of oxygenated air. Although shallow breathing may feel "normal," it can make you feel short of breath and anxious. Conversely, deep abdominal breathing encourages the full exchange of oxygen, creating a beneficial trade-off of incoming oxygen for outgoing carbon dioxide. As a result, it lowers or stabilizes blood pressure and slows heart rate.

For a small number of people, breathing exercises can increase anxiety, especially if they aren't practiced correctly. It's important to never force an inhalation or exhalation or try to control your breath. Instead, let your breath come and go naturally. The idea is to simply *observe* your natural breath and slowly count along with it. Trying to create an unnatural breathing pattern will promote stress and tension, which defeats the purpose of the exercise. Just relax, let your breath flow automatically, and watch it in your mind's eye.

To practice deep breathing, first find a quiet, comfortable place to sit or lie down. Rest your hands comfortably in your lap, or if you're lying down, let your arms relax beside your body. Alternatively, put both hands on your tummy, covering your belly button. Breathe in slowly through your nose to a count of 5, allowing your lower belly to rise as you fill your lungs. Let your inhalation completely fill your lungs, gently and naturally expanding your lower abdomen, not your chest. Now breathe out slowly through your mouth or your nose (if that feels more comfortable) to a count of 8 or 10. Completely release the air during your exhalation, letting the abdomen relax and naturally retract. If your hands are on your tummy, they should rise and fall along with your breath.

Establish a regular practice of deep breathing for 5 to 10 minutes once or twice day, preferably at the same time every day. As you sit comfortably with your eyes closed, blend deep breathing with calming imagery or focus on a word or phrase that helps you relax, or simply count slowly to 5 with your inhalation and count slowly to 8 or 10 with your exhalation.

MINDFULNESS-BASED STRESS REDUCTION

Mindfulness-Based Stress Reduction (MBSR) is a formal eight-week group program that was developed by Jon Kabat-Zinn in the 1970s to treat patients struggling with life's difficulties or with physical and/or mental illness. Although it was initially created to aid hospital patients, it has wide applicability and has been used by a broad range of people from all walks of life. Currently the program is in over 250 hospitals around the United States and many more around the world. Most MBSR classes for patients are taught by physicians, nurses, psychologists, and social workers, as well as other health professionals.

At the core of MBSR is the practice of mindfulness, which involves focusing your attention on one thing in the moment, whether it's each breath you take, each step as you walk, or the sights or sounds around you. The program challenges participants to practice present-moment awareness, deep relaxation, and gentle movement. Through the use of these techniques, participants learn to discover and observe their reactions to life's stressors so they can consciously choose how to respond. With practice, they can then apply these skills to everyday situations.

MBSR can help people who are coping with medical problems, job or family-related stress, anxiety, or depression. Most participants report lasting decreases in both physical and psychological symptoms, with reduced pain levels or better coping skills for chronic pain. The majority of people also report an increased ability to relax, greater enthusiasm for life, enhanced self-esteem, and improved ability to deal more effectively with stressful situations.

PROGRESSIVE MUSCLE RELAXATION

Progressive muscle relaxation (PMR) is a technique that focuses on relaxing each individual muscle group. It's often combined with deep breathing (see page 102) and is simple to learn. Although it's helpful anytime you feel stressed, it's especially useful for promoting sleep, so you might want to do PMR at bedtime. Practicing PMR regularly will make it much more effective and produce a relaxed mental and physical state more rapidly.

To begin, move to a quiet room that's warm but not excessively warm. Make sure you won't be interrupted by other people or the phone, computer, or doorbell. Lie down with your arms and legs uncrossed. Close your eyes and take a deep breath through your nose to a count of 4, hold it for a count of 4, then exhale slowly through your mouth or nose to a count of 8. Repeat three more times. Maintain a slow, deep breathing pattern throughout the entire exercise.

Now concentrate on each part of the body, beginning with the top of your head and progressing downward. Be sure to include the scalp, forehead, ears, eyes, eyelids, mouth, front of the neck, back of the neck, shoulders, upper back, lower back, arms, hands, fingers, chest, belly, buttocks, thighs, calves, feet, toes, and bottoms of the feet. Some people prefer to go in the opposite direction, from the bottoms of the feet to the top of the head. Choose which direction you prefer most and then stick with it.

To further increase your awareness and relaxation, tense each muscle as tightly as possible for a count of 5 to 10, and then release it completely. Experience the muscle as totally relaxed and as heavy as lead. It should feel as though it's sinking deep into the floor or bed. Feel the muscles relax and become loose and limp, with tension flowing out of them like water from a faucet. Focus on and notice the difference between the sensation of tension and relaxation. Let your whole body and all your cells relax and feel warm and comfortable.

VISUALIZATION

Visualization is a technique in which you form mental images to take a visual journey to a calming place or situation that makes you feel happy, relaxed, and peaceful. Visualization differs somewhat from other stress-management exercises because it involves the senses. To relax using visualization, try to incorporate as many senses as possible, including sight, smell, sound, and touch. For example, if you imagine relaxing in a garden or at a park on a sunny day, think about the smell of the grass and flowers, the sound of a nearby burbling brook, and the warmth of the sun on your face. If you imagine relaxing at the ocean, think about the smell of salt water, the sound of crashing waves, and the feeling of sinking into the warm, sandy beach. To begin, sit or lie down in a quiet, comfortable place where you won't be disturbed. Loosen any tight clothing, close your eyes, and concentrate on your breathing as you focus on positive images, experiences, and thoughts.

There are a few other ways that you can use visualization to help you relax. For instance, you could create mental images of stress flowing out of your body, or of your problems, worries, concerns, or distractions melting into the ground or being folded up and stashed away in a padlocked box.

SELF-HYPNOSIS

One of the principal tenets of hypnosis is inducing a deeply relaxed state, which makes it an ideal tool for both reducing and managing stress. Although you certainly could visit a hypnotherapist or listen to hypnosis CDs (both of which may be worthwhile for you to explore!), you can also learn some easy and effective self-hypnosis techniques to relieve stress. You only need to practice self-hypnosis a few minutes each day or several times a week to help reduce the negative effects of stress on your life and health.

If you like, you can include one or more affirmations (see box, opposite page) during your self-hypnosis sessions. Affirmations are specific positive statements to help you visualize and believe what you're affirming so you can overcome negative, self-sabotaging thoughts. Write down your affirmations in advance of each session, and try to make them goal-oriented so they meet your objectives. For instance, if you want to lessen your anxiety around other people, you could create an affirmation such as "I feel safe, calm, and peaceful wherever I am" or "I am confident and self-assured." Always keep your affirmations in the present tense.

Once you have decided on which affirmations to use, find a quiet, private place free of any distractions. Get in a comfortable sitting position that will allow you to easily relax. Don't lie down, however, as that will make it too easy to fall asleep, especially if you are tired.

In order for hypnosis to be effective, it's important to be deeply relaxed. Close your eyes and do some slow, deep breathing (see page 102). Silently repeat helpful statements to yourself that will encourage letting go and relaxing, such as "I feel the tension flowing out of my body with each exhalation" or "I am becoming increasingly relaxed with every breath." Continue to breathe slowly and deeply. You can also do progressive muscle relaxation (see page 104) as well as picture the stress flowing out of your body.

Visualization (see page 105) can play a valuable role in self-hypnosis. Imagine a place you associate with positive feelings, such as a beautiful garden filled with flowers, a lush forest, or a sandy beach.

Picture yourself in this serene, tranquil place. After several minutes of practicing deep breathing, progressive muscle relaxation, and visualization, you should feel very relaxed. Now you can begin to repeat the affirmations you created for this particular session. If you choose not to use affirmations, simply envision yourself calm, relaxed, and worry-free. Focus your mind on this image or on your affirmation. If you prefer, you can tape both the relaxation statements and your affirmations in advance so you can simply focus on the sound of your voice, just as you would if you were in a session with a hypnotherapist.

Experiment with different places, positions, or techniques to enhance your self-hypnosis sessions and discover what works best for you. Although results won't happen overnight and may be subtle or incremental, if you practice self-hypnosis regularly, you should find that it has a positive effect on your stress levels and overall sense of well-being.

Sample Affirmations FOR RELIEF OF STRESS, ANXIETY, AND PAIN

I accept myself just as I am.

I am at peace with my past, present, and future.

I am calm and centered.

I am courageous and strong.

I am safe and protected.

I fill my mind with positive, nourishing thoughts.

I inhale confidence. I exhale fear.

I send love and healing to every organ of my body.

I trust my inner wisdom.

My cells vibrate with energy and health.

My mind is quiet and serene.

My presence is my power.

POSITIVE SELF-TALK

We all have a set of messages that our minds play over and over again. Too often this internal discourse is negative. We remember the admonitions of parents, teachers, bosses, siblings, and peers, and as we replay them, they fuel our feelings of anger, guilt, fear, helplessness, and hopelessness. One of the most effective ways to overcome these self-sabotaging messages is to "overwrite" them with positive self-talk.

To do that, first write down some of the negative messages that plague you the most. Now counteract those negative messages with positive truths about yourself and your life. If a positive truth doesn't come to mind immediately, keep thinking until you find one. For every negative message there's a positive truth that overrides it. For example, you may have a negative message that replays in your head every time you make a mistake, such as "You never do anything right" or "You'll never amount to anything." When you make a mistake, you can choose to overwrite that message with a positive statement, such as "As I learn from my mistakes, I become a better person" or "I accept my mistakes and grow from them." When you feel worried, agitated, or on edge, your mind may play another critical message from your past, such as "You're a nervous wreck" or "You always fall apart." You can shift that destructive chatter to something constructive and heartening, such as "I'm strong; I can handle this" or "I have the power to stop what I don't want."

Note that this isn't self-deception. Positive self-talk encourages acknowledgment of the many favorable qualities and truths about yourself (and your life, and life in general) that are often obscured or suppressed. By engaging positive self-talk, you can focus on your strengths, lift yourself up, and remain calm in any given situation.

MASSAGE THERAPY

Massage not only feels great, but it has also been shown to be effective in reducing perceived stress and anxiety levels. However, there are several different forms of massage, and although some are relaxing, others may be more stimulating and invigorating. Moderate pressure, as with Swedish massage, tends to lower blood pressure and enhance relaxation, while trigger point therapy and deep tissue massage may actually raise blood pressure. Try different types of massage to find the ones that feel best to you and that make you feel the most relaxed.

Some forms of massage can cause a little muscle soreness the following day, but for the most part, massage shouldn't be painful or uncomfortable. If at any time during your session you feel pain or discomfort, let your massage therapist know immediately.

Although most people can benefit from massage, it may not be suitable for individuals with certain health conditions, especially pregnant women and people with cancer, fractures, or unexplained pain. If you have any concerns, talk with your health provider in advance about whether massage is appropriate for you.

MEDITATION

Meditation has been practiced for thousands of years. Originally intended to deepen human understanding of the esoteric and sacred forces of life, it's primarily used today to produce a deep state of relaxation and a tranquil mind. Meditation involves focused attention, which helps to eliminate the constant mental chatter that jumbles our thoughts and causes stress. It's simple and inexpensive and doesn't require any special clothing or equipment. It also can be practiced by anyone, regardless of age or health. You can meditate wherever you find yourself: stuck in traffic, standing in line at the supermarket, riding the bus, out for a walk, waiting at the doctor's office, or even in challenging social settings or business meetings.

Meditation can impart a sense of calm, peace, and balance that can benefit emotional well-being as well as overall health. These benefits are far-reaching and continue long after the meditation session ends. In rare cases meditation can worsen symptoms associated with certain mental health conditions, particularly in people with psychosis, for whom meditating may trigger a psychotic event. Talk with your health-care provider before embarking on a meditation practice if you have any concerns.

Some experts recommend meditating for no longer than twenty minutes in the morning after waking up and then again in the early evening before dinner, although others favor longer sessions. Even meditating just once a day for a few minutes can be helpful. New practitioners should be aware that it can be difficult to quiet the mind, so don't be discouraged if you don't experience immediate results. A few of the most common features and types of meditation include the following:

Focused attention. Focusing your attention is perhaps the most important and defining element of meditation, and it's what helps free the mind from the many distractions that contribute to stress and worry. You can focus your attention on a specific object, an image, a mantra (see page 112), or your breathing (see "Deep Breathing," page 102, and "Conscious Breathing," page 13).

A quiet setting. If you're just starting out with meditation, you may find it will be easier if you're in a quiet location with no distractions (including no music, talking, noise, or electronics). As you become more skilled, you may be able to meditate almost anywhere, even in high-stress situations where it can be very beneficial, such as a difficult or demanding work meeting, a long line at the grocery store, or a traffic jam.

Diaphragmatic breathing. Also called deep breathing, abdominal breathing, belly breathing, and several other names, this technique involves deep, even-paced breaths that use the diaphragm to expand the lungs. The diaphragm is a large, dome-shaped muscle located at the base of the lungs. This technique will slow down your breathing and help you take in more oxygen. To learn diaphragmatic breathing, see "Deep Breathing," page 102, and "Conscious Breathing," page 13.

A comfortable position. Meditation can be practiced sitting, lying down, walking, or when you're in other positions or doing other activities. The important thing to bear in mind is that you should be comfortable so you can get the most out of your meditation session. Strive to maintain good posture throughout the entire meditation.

Stay open. Let your thoughts, emotions, and physical sensations pass through your mind without judgment. It's common for the mind to wander during meditation, regardless of how long a person has been been practicing meditation. If your attention wanders, gently return your attention to the focus of your meditation (such as your breath or mantra).

Don't let the idea of meditating the "right" way add to your stress. If you like, you can take a meditation class led by a trained instructor, but it's just as easy to learn and practice meditation on your own. Meditation can suit your lifestyle or situation, and you can make it as formal and structured or informal and "casual" as you like. For instance, some people start each day with twenty minutes to an hour of meditation, often before sunup, or meditate just before bedtime, while others simply slip in a few minutes of quality meditation at various times throughout the day.

Meditation is essentially an umbrella term that encompasses a wide number of techniques used to achieve a relaxed state of mind. In fact, many of the exercises listed in this section could fall under the category of meditation because they all share the same core objective of helping the practitioner achieve calm and serenity. For example, guided meditation is the same as visualization (see page 105), also known as guided imagery. Self-hypnosis (see page 106), deep breathing (see page 102), conscious breathing (see page 13), and even progressive muscle relaxation (see page 104) could fall under the heading of meditation. Experiment to find the types of meditation that work best for you and that you enjoy, and adapt the meditation to your needs at that moment. There's no right or wrong way to meditate. What's important is that your meditation helps you to reduce stress and feel better overall. Here are a few additional types of meditation you might want to try:

Body scanning. When using this meditation technique, focus your attention on different parts of your body. Become aware of the body's various sensations, such as tension, pain, warmth, or relaxation. You can combine body scanning with breathing exercises, such as breathing heat or relaxation into and out of different parts of your body.

Mantra meditation. The essence of the word "mantra" is the sum of its two parts: "man," which means "mind," and "tra," which means "transport" or "vehicle." This "mind vehicle" is actually a powerful tool in the form of a sound, word, or phrase that is silently repeated to prevent distracting thoughts and help the mind enter a deep state of peace and relaxation. Chanting (see page 15) is another form of mantra meditation, but with chanting the mantra is spoken aloud.

You can create your own mantra, whether it's secular or spiritually based. Mantras don't need to have any special meaning attached to them to work. A number of common mantras are in other languages that the practitioner may not even understand, or they are simply special sounds, and yet they still are quite effective in terms of keeping the brain focused. Some groups encourage using mantras that have personal significance for the practitioner, and in that way they can then be used similarly to affirmations (see page 107).

You could select a simple one-word mantra, such as "relax," "serenity," "love," "kindness," "patience," or "peace." Alternatively, you could use something more spiritual in nature, such as "OM," which is derived from ancient Sanskrit. The yogic mantra "So-Hum" is a reflection of the sound of the breath, but it also carries a contemplative meaning: "I am that" ("so" means "I am," and "hum" means "that"). In this usage, "that" refers to all of creation—the one breathing us all. When practicing the So-Hum mantra, inhale slowly and deeply through your nose while silently saying the word "so." Then slowly exhale through your nose while silently saying the word "hum," extending the "mmm" sound in your mind. Continue to silently repeat "so . . . hum" with each inhalation and exhalation. Alternatively, silently say the full mantra ("so-hum") as you slowly and deeply inhale, and repeat it silently again as you slowly and fully exhale, extending the "mmm" sound in your mind with each exhalation.

Try to coordinate deep breathing (see page 102) in conjunction with your mantra throughout your meditation. Very short mantras (two to five syllables) can be used with the out-breath only, if you prefer, with no mantra used for the in-breath. At the end of your meditation, rest in silence for a few minutes before slowly standing and gradually returning to the activities of your daily life.

Here are a few more short mantras you can try:

- Breathing in, I am calm. Breathing out, I am free.
- Everything I need is within me.
- I accept what is. I let go of what was.
- I am that I am.
- Let it be. Let it go.
- Inhale wisdom. Exhale tension.
- It is what it is.
- May I be happy. May I be free.
- Surrender. Release.
- This too shall pass.

You may also want to try memorizing and silently reciting and repeating one (or two or all) of the following short poems for your meditation:

> May I be free from fear.
> May I be free from suffering.
> May I be happy and well.
> May I be filled with peace.

> Peace is above me
> Peace is below me.
> Peace is before me.
> Peace is behind me.
> Peace is within me.
> Peace is all around me.

Health, fill my body.
Health, fill my mind.
Health, fill my spirit.
Health, fill my actions.
Health, fill my choices.
Health, fill my heart.

I act with courage.
I am safe from harm.
My fears are diminished.
My spirit is healed.

I am grateful for today.
I am hopeful for tomorrow.
I do my best in all things.
I honor my journey by living in peace.
I honor my journey by releasing the past.
I honor my journey by taking care of my health.
I honor my journey by dwelling in the present.
I honor my journey by loving who I am.

May my spirit be open and accepting.
May kindness grow within me.
May I have the courage to accept my limitations.
May I be patient with myself and others.

My strength is equal to my challenges.

I trust my skills and abilities.

I trust my experience and wisdom.

I am confident and capable.

Mindfulness meditation. This type of meditation is based on being mindful, which means having an increased awareness and acceptance of living in or being in the present moment. When you practice mindfulness meditation, you focus on what you are experiencing during the meditation, such as the flow of your breath. Many other types of meditation use similar techniques.

To begin, sit upright with your spine straight, either cross-legged (on a blanket or special meditation cushion) or sitting on a firm chair with both feet on the floor, uncrossed. Rest your hands comfortably in your lap with the palms facing up, one on top of the other. With your eyes closed or gently looking a few feet ahead of you, observe the inhalation and exhalation of your breath. As your mind wanders, simply note it as a fact and return your attention to your breath. Notice the coolness of the in-breath and the warmth of the out-breath at the edges of your nostrils. As you observe your thoughts, physical sensations, and emotions, let them pass without judgment, like clouds floating by, and again return your focus to your breath.

Passage meditation. This type of meditation is similar to silent mantra meditation (see page 112) and entails silently repeating memorized poems or portions of sacred texts. If you like, try using one or more of the short poems on pages 113–115 for this meditation.

Prayer meditation. Prayer is perhaps the best known and most widely practiced example of meditation. Spoken and written prayers are found in most spiritual traditions. You can pray using your own words or by reading prayers written by others.

Walking meditation. An efficient and healthy way to relax is by meditating while you walk. You can use this technique anywhere you're walking, whether you're in a tranquil forest, at the beach, on a city sidewalk, or at the mall. Don't be concerned about a destination. Instead, slow down your pace so you can focus on the movement of your legs or feet. If you like, you can silently repeat words that describe the actions of your body, such as "lifting," "moving," and "placing" as you lift each foot, move your leg forward, and place your foot on the ground.

The following practices are generally considered forms of "meditation in motion" or "movement meditation." They differ from the conventional notion of meditation in that instead of the body being stationary, specific movements are coordinated with the breath and with focused attention.

Qi gong. Pronounced CHEE-gung, this practice is part of traditional Chinese medicine. It combines meditation, relaxation, physical movement, and breathing exercises to help restore and maintain balance along with physical and mental health.

Tai chi. Pronounced TIE-CHEE, this tradition is a form of gentle Chinese martial arts. In tai chi you perform a self-paced series of postures or movements in a slow, graceful manner while practicing deep breathing.

Yoga. In this ancient Indian practice, a series of postures and controlled breathing exercises are performed to promote a more flexible body and a calm mind. As you move through poses that require balance and concentration, you're encouraged to focus on the present moment.

Diet

A diet high in stress-inducing chemicals, sugars, and refined carbohydrates can negatively affect the adrenal glands, disrupt sleep and hormone function, and adversely influence weight and mood. Stress promotes greater physiologic demands, so it's not surprising that we require a more nutrient-dense diet during periods of stress. Ironically, however, stress can cause unhealthy eating habits.

When people have chronic stress, they often have little time to fit a balanced diet into their busy schedules. Many individuals turn to fast foods and comfort foods that are high in fat, sugar, and salt and lacking the essential vitamins and minerals their bodies need to deal with stressful circumstances. In addition, when people are stressed or not feeling well, they may skip meals or forget to eat. These dietary insufficiencies can lead to nutritional deficiencies that put an even greater burden on the body, which further compromises metabolic systems and poses a threat to both physical and mental health.

Because people enduring stress are frequently tired, even to the point of exhaustion, they may use coffee or other stimulants to give them a boost of energy and help them cope. But products that contain caffeine, especially in large quantities, can have adverse effects on the body and mind. People who rely on caffeine to stay awake undermine the rest their bodies desperately need and disrupt their natural circadian sleep cycle. Caffeine increases the production of certain hormones in the body, such as adrenaline and cortisol, as well as the neurotransmitter dopamine, which is a precursor of epinephrine. The increased amount of cortisol produced by stress further contributes to the urge to eat foods high in refined carbohydrates, sugars, and fats. Nutritional deficiencies often lead to chronic physical and emotional problems, such as lethargy, lapses in concentration, and mood swings. If the nutritional consequences of stress aren't properly dealt with, the body could suffer serious, long-term health repercussions, such as diabetes, high blood pressure, and high cholesterol.

Although some websites and alternative practitioners specializing in "adrenal fatigue" may advise eating or avoiding certain foods at particular times of the day, there isn't any scientific evidence to support these suggestions. A special "adrenal fatigue diet" and treatment protocol may help improve an individual's health, but that's only because it encourages important diet and lifestyle improvements rather than directly providing a boost to adrenal gland function. The basic diet for "adrenal fatigue" is comparable to any diet for a healthy lifestyle: eat at regular intervals every day and have meals that are based on low-fat, high-fiber, carbohydrate-rich whole foods, such as whole grains, starchy and non-starchy vegetables, and fresh fruits. These foods will soothe and nourish the body, impart energy naturally, and provide the nutrients you need to bolster your immune system and all the systems of your body. Depriving yourself of these foods, however, will leave you feeling tired and fatigued all day long. The carbohydrates found in whole grains are released slowly into the bloodstream, so a diet centered around unrefined whole grains helps thwart the typical energy "crash" that occurs with the consumption of caffeine, chocolate, or sugar. Eating whole grains will help you maintain a steady level of energy throughout the day and won't leave you with an afternoon slump.

Certain whole foods that are naturally high in carbohydrates, such as bananas, brown rice, oatmeal, pumpkins, and sweet potatoes, contain large amounts of tryptophan, an amino acid that helps relax the body and aids sleep. Brown rice, oatmeal, polenta, tart cherries, and walnuts are just some of the many wholesome foods that contain melatonin, the hormone that regulates sleep. Eating a small amount of foods rich in complex carbohydrates a few hours before bedtime will help you fall asleep more quickly and will keep you sleeping more soundly through the night.

All whole-food sources of carbohydrates are also excellent sources of fiber. Fiber regulates digestion, facilitates proper bowel function, and keeps glycemic levels steady so you can stay satisfied longer and won't get hungry quite as quickly. Unlike sugar and caffeine, which cause anxiety and jitteriness, complex carbohydrates provide a grounding effect that reduces anxiety and provides the balance and sustenance your body needs during times of stress.

Avoid refined carbohydrates, such as white flour, sugar of any kind (including "healthy" sugars, such as agave nectar, brown rice syrup, brown sugar, honey, maple syrup, and molasses), and breads, rolls, cereals, and other processed foods that contain refined grains or sugars. The tips in the sections that follow will help you make the best choices.

FOODS THAT RELIEVE STRESS AND PROMOTE RELAXATION

Scientists believe that complex carbohydrates cause the brain to produce more serotonin, a hormone that aids relaxation, improves mood, and promotes healthy sleep patterns. High-fiber foods increase satiety, support healthy bowel function, and can help thwart potentially harmful food cravings. The following are a few of the many foods that fall into this category:

- legumes (beans, lentils, peas)
- oatmeal
- sweet potatoes and yams
- white potatoes with skin
- whole grains (such as brown rice, bulgur, millet, and quinoa)
- winter squash

Chronic stress can weaken the immune system and impede our ability to fight disease. Increasing our intake of antioxidant-rich fruits and vegetables can reverse this process by boosting the immune system. By simply choosing from a wide array of deeply colored fruits and veggies (such as beets, berries, cherries, melons, peppers, and dark leafy greens), you can readily find the ones that are highest in antioxidants.

FOODS THAT EXACERBATE STRESS

Foods that are high in fat, particularly animal fat (such as meat, cheese, and butter), elevate blood pressure, make our blood thick and sticky, and cause us to feel tired and sluggish. As a result, fatty, high-cholesterol foods contribute to weight gain, depression, and lethargy, as well as increase the risk of heart attack.

Although small amounts of caffeine can provide a short-term energy boost and temporarily elevate mood, too much caffeine increases cortisol secretion, raises blood pressure, causes tension and jitteriness, interferes with sleep, and can make people feel stressed even if they weren't to begin with. Drinking caffeinated beverages (coffee, tea, cola) will exacerbate stress, not alleviate it. While it's true that weaning yourself off caffeine can be rough for a few days, it will be beneficial to your long-term stress reduction.

Because sugar is a carbohydrate, it can initially impart a sense of calm. But since it's a simple carbohydrate, it enters and leaves the bloodstream rapidly, causing an energy "rush" followed by a nasty "crash," ultimately creating a vicious up-down cycle that can leave you feeling irritable and drained. It's best to avoid all types of sugar and other simple carbohydrate foods, such as candy, desserts, pastries, sodas, syrups, and white bread.

Many people are under the false impression that alcohol is a relaxant, and they therefore think it's okay to imbibe during periods of stress. While a small glass of wine or a shot of whiskey might provide some short-term relief, in the long run it can do more harm than good. Alcohol damages the liver and depresses adrenal function, and although reduced cortisol production may initially seem like a good thing, over time it can impair the immune system, increase inflammation, and disrupt healthy sleep patterns. To lower stress levels and improve overall health, it's best to avoid alcohol consumption completely.

CULINARY HERBS AND SPICES

Although you're no doubt aware that herbs and spices taste great, you may be surprised to learn that many of them can also help the body cope with acute or chronic stress. In addition, they can help support and strengthen the immune system when the adrenal glands are overwhelmed. Some of the best options are cardamom, cinnamon, cloves, coriander, fennel seeds, garlic, ginger, oregano, peppermint, spearmint, thyme, and turmeric. If you have access to fresh herbs, such as basil, cilantro, dill, mint, oregano, sage, or thyme, all the better. Incorporate these herbs and spices regularly in your meals by adding them to recipes or sprinkling them over finished dishes, whole grains, vegetables, and salads. They will not only help boost your general health but will also elevate the flavor of your food considerably. Alternatively, enjoy these flavorful herbs and spices in the form of herbal teas.

ADDITIONAL TIPS

Your body needs fuel at regular intervals throughout the day. Honor that need by giving it real (rather than refined and processed) foods on a consistent basis. Avoid skipping meals, especially breakfast and lunch, as that will result in an unwelcome drop in blood sugar later in the day, along with elevated stress levels.

While it's important to have regularly scheduled meals, monitor your portion sizes. Overeating puts undue stress on the body and slows down digestion, which can make you feel even more sluggish. Eat at a relaxed pace, not on the run or in the car. Choose a calm environment, such as a quiet spot in a park or cafe when you're not at home. Eat mindfully and avoid eating while watching TV or surfing the web; focus on your food instead. Mindful eating will support your adrenals and digestion, lower your stress levels, and make it easier to stop when you're satisfied so you don't overeat.

Finally, avoid eating right before you go to bed. It takes about three hours for food to be fully processed and digested after you eat, and the body can't properly rest and digest food simultaneously. Either rest or digestion or both will suffer if you go to bed directly after a meal, putting an unnecessary strain on the body. While foods high in complex carbohydrates can help you fall asleep and will promote more sustained sleep, enjoy them a few hours prior to bedtime.

Vitamins and Minerals

Poor eating and lifestyle habits as a result of stress can take a terrible toll on nutritional intakes, further burdening the body's systems. When stress overtakes your life, there are a few nutrients in particular that you should pay special attention to. While most of these can be obtained through diet, a few will require supplementation.

B-complex vitamins help with nervous system functioning, and experiencing severe or ongoing stress can deplete your levels. Vitamin B_{12} and other B vitamins play a vital role in producing brain chemicals that affect anxiety and mood and certain brain functions. Low levels of B_{12} and other B vitamins, such as vitamin B_6 and folate, are linked to low energy, fuzzy thinking, poor stress response, and possibly depression. Try to obtain your B vitamins from whole foods (such as almonds, beans, berries, broccoli, dark leafy greens, dried fruits, and fortified nondairy milks and yogurts), but take a B-complex supplement or multivitamin-mineral supplement if you feel your diet is lacking. Almost everyone should supplement with sublingual vitamin B_{12}, which isn't found in sufficient quantities in food to ensure the daily recommended amount. This nutrient is essential to healthy hormones, brain and nervous system function, red blood cell production, and overall health, so supplementing with it, especially for older individuals and anyone under stress, is essential. The urinary methylmalonic acid (uMMA) test for vitamin B_{12} reflects tissue/cellular deficiency, and for that reason it is far more accurate than a blood test. The uMMA assay is considered the gold standard for identifying tissue B_{12} deficiency, so be sure to ask your health-care provider to order a uMMA test for you rather than the standard blood test used to check B_{12} levels.

Magnesium plays a role in over three hundred of the body's biochemical reactions and regulates the release of stress hormones. Research has shown a strong connection between low magnesium levels and depression and anxiety. Magnesium-rich foods include dark-green leafy vegetables (such as chard, kale, and spinach), as well as avocados, bananas, dark chocolate, figs, legumes (beans, lentils, and peas), nuts (especially almonds, Brazil nuts, and cashews), seeds (especially pumpkin seeds), tofu, and whole grains.

Tryptophan isn't a vitamin or mineral but rather an essential amino acid. It's the leading supplement purchased for stress and anxiety. Tryptophan converts into a compound called 5-HTP, which then converts to serotonin (the "feel good" chemical), which plays an important role in regulating appetite, mood, and sleep. Although all high-protein foods contain tryptophan, that doesn't mean the body can use the tryptophan from those protein sources. For example, cow's milk contains a good amount of tryptophan, but it also is abundant in pro-inflammatory cytokines that will degrade tryptophan. Furthermore, animal-based proteins are loaded with saturated fat and lack fiber and vitamin C, which makes it difficult for the body to use tryptophan for the production of serotonin and melatonin. Surprisingly, some of the best tryptophan-containing foods are plant-based. Unlike animal products, plants are rich in health-supporting anti-inflammatory fats, fiber, and antioxidants, and many of them also contain the tryptophan cofactors vitamin B_6, vitamin C, folic acid, and magnesium. Good plant-based sources of trypto-phan include bananas, dark leafy greens, legumes (beans, lentils, and peas), nuts (especially walnuts), potatoes, seeds (especially pumpkin seeds), soy products (edamame, soy milk, tempeh, tofu), spirulina, whole grains (oats, quinoa, whole wheat), and winter squashes.

Vitamin D is known as the "sunshine vitamin" because its main source is sunlight. People who live in climates with cold, dark winters are at significantly higher risk for deficiency, although it's estimated that 30–100 percent of all people are deficient in vitamin D! Research has confirmed that individuals with depression and anxiety disorders commonly have low levels of this nutrient. Fortified foods (such as fortified juices and nondairy milks) may contain a measure of vita-min D, but if you have darker skin, don't spend much time outdoors, or are an older adult, vitamin D supplementation is critical to ensure you're getting adequate amounts.

Calcium deficiency is less common than a deficiency in magne-sium or vitamins B_{12} or D, but it can nevertheless have a powerful effect on mental and physical health. The nervous system requires cal-cium to function properly, so mood disorders and anxiety often arise with insufficient calcium intakes. The physical symptoms of calcium deficiency include tingling sensations, numbness, shaking, and heart palpitations, which are also common physical symptoms of anxiety. Calcium-rich food choices include almonds, dark-green leafy vegeta-bles, oatmeal, fortified nondairy milks, and fortified soy products.

Everyone should have a yearly physical exam that includes test-ing for vitamin and mineral levels. Some people, especially those who are deficient in certain nutrients (such as vitamin B_{12} or vitamin D) may need to be tested more frequently. Be sure to speak with your health-care provider before starting a new supplement regimen.

Herbal and Natural Remedies

Because people who experience symptoms associated with "adrenal fatigue" are desperate for solutions, they are often motivated to explore herbal and other natural remedies. Although many benefits have been attributed to these remedies, few, if any, have scientific support. In addition, just as with standard drugs, these so-called natural remedies can have side effects and may cause health problems, some of which could be serious. Similarly, homeopathic remedies have not shown to be effective treatments.

In general, manufacturers of herbal remedies and dietary supplements don't need approval of the US Food and Drug Administration (FDA) to sell their products. However, herbs and supplements can affect the body's chemistry in the same way that pharmaceuticals can, and they therefore have the potential to produce side effects that may be harmful or even lethal. Always check with your doctor or health-care provider before using any herbal remedies or dietary supplements, and be wary of any product that promises a quick cure or that requires the purchase of expensive treatments. These treatments may be useless, and therefore a waste of money, but even worse, they might be dangerous.

Conclusion

If you have been to the doctor for your symptoms, gone through multiple diagnostic tests that have come back negative, and been told there's nothing medically wrong with you, it's time to employ a different strategy. The solution to feeling better is actually close at hand. With the guidance outlined in this chapter and throughout this book, you can begin to identify the lifestyle patterns and behaviors you're engaging in that are causing your body to be under constant strain and consequently compromising your health. It's crucial to recognize the importance of the lifestyle changes that are readily available to you and that can reduce or eliminate your symptoms.

The effects that stress can have on a person's health are serious and can wreak havoc with every major system of the body, resulting in the cluster of symptoms often referred to as "adrenal fatigue." But with the right approaches, you can minimize the impact stress has on your body and effectively repair and reverse any damage that has been done. Wise behavioral choices and a healthy lifestyle are essential companions to any stress-reduction program. The antidote is directly within your reach.

GLOSSARY

Adaptation. The physiological changes that take place as a result of the body's response to a stressor.

Adrenal cortex. The outer portion of the adrenal glands. The adrenal cortex produces two main groups of corticosteroid hormones—glucocorticoids and mineralocorticoids—that are essential to life.

Adrenal medulla. The inner portion of the adrenal glands. The adrenal medulla produces several "stress hormones," including epinephrine (adrenaline) and norepinephrine (noradrenaline).

Allostasis. The process by which a state of internal, physiological balance (homeostasis) is maintained in response to actual or perceived environmental and psychological stressors.

Autonomic nervous system. A part of the nervous system that regulates key involuntary functions of the body, including the activity of the heart muscle, the glands, and the smooth muscles, including the muscles of the intestinal tract. The autonomic nervous system has two divisions: (1) the sympathetic nervous system, which accelerates heart rate, constricts blood vessels, and raises blood pressure, and (2) the parasympathetic nervous system, which slows heart rate, increases intestinal and gland activity, and relaxes the sphincter muscles.

Coping. The balancing act between biological, psychological, and social processes in response to acute or chronic stress.

Cytokines. Any of a number of immunoregulatory proteins (such as interferon, interleukin, and growth factors) that are secreted by certain cells of the immune system and that have an effect on other cells.

Disease. A pathophysiological response to internal or external factors with an established biological cause, a defined group of symptoms, and a consistent change in bodily structure due to the condition, which isn't a result of physical injury.

Disorder. A cluster of symptoms that disrupt regular bodily structure and/or function that are not accounted for by a more pervasive condition and have no implication of etiology.

Distress or negative stress. Uncontrollable, prolonged, or overwhelming stress that is destructive.

Endocrinologists. Medical doctors who specialize in hormone-related health problems.

Etiology. The cause, set of causes, or manner of causation of a disease or condition.

Eustress. Also called "positive stress." Manageable stress that can lead to growth and enhanced competence.

Functional. Affecting the operation, rather than the structure, of an organ.

Glucocorticoids. A class of steroid hormones produced by the adrenal glands that are known particularly for their anti-inflammatory and immunosuppressive actions. Together with mineralocorticoids, glucocorticoids are used in replacement therapy to treat acute adrenal insufficiency (adrenal crisis) or chronic adrenal insufficiency (Addison's disease).

Homeostasis. The tendency of biological systems to maintain relatively constant conditions in the internal environment while continuously interacting with and adjusting to changes originating within or outside the system. Homeostasis literally means "same state."

HPA axis. The hypothalamic-pituitary-adrenal (HPA) axis is an interactive neuroendocrine unit composed of the hypothalamus (H), the pituitary gland (P), and the adrenal glands (A). The HPA axis plays key roles in basal homeostasis and in the body's response to stress.

Hyperarousal. An abnormal state of heightened responsiveness to stimuli that results in physiological manifestations, such as insomnia, irritability, impaired concentration, hypervigilance, and increased startle reactions.

Hypothalamus. A small area in the center of the brain that's responsible for maintaining the body's internal balance (homeostasis). It plays an important role in hormone production and helps to stimulate many important processes in the body (such as heart rate, blood pressure, electrolyte balance, appetite, body weight, sleep cycles, and glandular secretions of the stomach and intestines) by influencing both the endocrine and nervous systems.

Mineralocorticoids. A class of steroid hormones secreted by the adrenal cortex that regulate and influence electrolyte metabolism (particularly sodium and potassium ions) and balance, which are functions essential to life. Aldosterone is the primary mineralocorticoid.

Neurobehavioral. A branch of science pertaining to the assessment of a person's nerve and brain function by studying his or her behavior.

Neurons. Specialized cells within the nervous system that transmit information over long distances within the body. A neuron receives electrical input signals from sensory cells (called sensory neurons) and from other neurons.

Neuropsychiatry. A branch of psychiatry that connects mental or emotional disturbances to disordered brain function.

Neurotransmitter. Also known as chemical messengers, neurotransmitters are brain chemicals that communicate information throughout the brain and body by relaying signals between nerve cells known as neurons. The brain uses neurotransmitters to tell the heart to beat, the lungs to breathe, and the stomach to digest.

Parasympathetic nervous system. The part of the autonomic nervous system that counterbalances the action of the sympathetic nerves and returns many physiological functions to normal levels. It controls homeostasis and the body at rest and is responsible for the body's "rest and digest" function.

Pathogenesis. The origin and manner of the development of a disease.

Pathognomonic marker. A distinguishing characteristic of a specific disease.

Pathophysiology. The functional changes that accompany a particular syndrome or disease.

Pituitary gland. A pea-sized organ located at the base of the brain that contains many regions with highly specialized functions. The pituitary gland is often called the master gland because it controls several other hormone glands in the body, including the thyroid, adrenals, ovaries, and testes. The hormones of the pituitary gland help regulate the functions of these other endocrine glands by sending signals to stimulate or inhibit their own hormone production. The functions of the hypothalamus and pituitary gland are closely intertwined, and the two are attached by a stalk known as the infundibulum.

Resilience. A resistant quality that allows a person to recovery quickly and thrive in spite of adversity.

Stress. The physiological, psychological, or emotional response of the human system to any demand for change.

Stressor. Anything that is perceived as challenging, threatening, or demanding.

Sympathetic nervous system. Part of the autonomic nervous system, which also includes the parasympathetic nervous system. Sympathetic nerves originate inside the vertebral column, toward the middle of the spinal cord, and serve to accelerate heart rate, constrict blood vessels, and raise blood pressure. Prolonged activation of the sympathetic nervous system elicits the release of adrenaline from the adrenal medulla, triggering what's commonly termed the fight-or-flight response.

Syndrome. A cluster of signs and symptoms that occur together and that characterize a particular abnormality or condition.

Thalamus. A small structure within the brain, located just above the brain stem between the cerebral cortex and the midbrain, with extensive nerve connections to both. The main function of the thalamus is to relay motor and sensory signals to the cerebral cortex. It also regulates sleep, alertness, and wakefulness.

RESOURCES

The American Institute of Stress

    stress.org

Cleveland Clinic Center
for Continuing Education/
Disease Management

    clevelandclinicmeded.com

Diet & Fitness Today

    dietandfitnesstoday.com

EndocrineWeb

    endocrineweb.com

Hormone Health Network

    hormone.org

Johns Hopkins Medicine
Health Library

    hopkinsmedicine.org

Medical News Today

    medicalnewstoday.com

Medline Plus

    medlineplus.gov

Medscape: Drugs & Diseases

    emedicine.medscape.com

National Adrenal Diseases
Foundation

    nadf.us

The National Center for
Biotechnology Information

    ncbi.nlm.nih.gov

The National Institute of Diabetes
and Digestive and Kidney Diseases

    niddk.nih.gov

Pituitary Network Association
Knowledge Base

    pituitary.org/knowledge-base

Science Daily

    sciencedaily.com

Science-Based Medicine

    sciencebasedmedicine.org

United States National Library
of Medicine, National Institutes
of Health

    https://www.nlm.nih.gov

INDEX

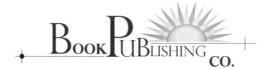

BookPublishing Co.

books that educate, inspire, and empower

Visit **BookPubCo.com** to find your favorite books on
plant-based cooking and nutrition, raw foods, and healthy living.

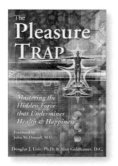

The Pleasure Trap
Douglas J. Lisle, PhD
Alan Goldhamer, DC
978-1-57067-197-5
$14.95

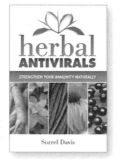

Herbal Antivirals
Sorrel Davis
978-1-57067-344-3
$12.95

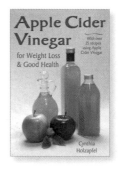

Apple Cider Vinegar
Cynthia Holzapfel
978-1-57067-127-2
$9.95

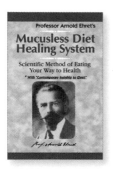

Mucusless Diet Healing
System
Arnold Ehret
978-1-88477-200-9
$9.95

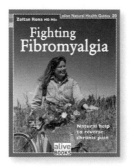

Fighting Fibromyalgia
Zoltan Rona, MD, MSc
978-1-55312-019-3
$11.95

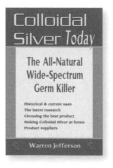

Colloidal Silver Today
Warren Jefferson
978-1-57067-154-8
$7.95

Purchase these titles from your favorite book source or buy them directly from:
Book Publishing Company • PO Box 99 • Summertown, TN 38483 • 1-888-260-8458

Free shipping and handling on all orders